Amal Khsiba
Moufida Mahmoudu
Lamine Hamzaoui

Digestive neuroendocrine tumors

Amal Khsiba
Moufida Mahmoudu
Lamine Hamzaoui

Digestive neuroendocrine tumors

ScienciaScripts

Imprint

Any brand names and product names mentioned in this book are subject to trademark, brand or patent protection and are trademarks or registered trademarks of their respective holders. The use of brand names, product names, common names, trade names, product descriptions etc. even without a particular marking in this work is in no way to be construed to mean that such names may be regarded as unrestricted in respect of trademark and brand protection legislation and could thus be used by anyone.

Cover image: www.ingimage.com

This book is a translation from the original published under ISBN 978-620-6-69324-6.

Publisher:
Sciencia Scripts
is a trademark of
Dodo Books Indian Ocean Ltd. and OmniScriptum S.R.L publishing group

120 High Road, East Finchley, London, N2 9ED, United Kingdom
Str. Armeneasca 28/1, office 1, Chisinau MD-2012, Republic of Moldova, Europe
Printed at: see last page
ISBN: 978-620-6-15752-6

Contents

I INTRODUCTION

Digestive neuroendocrine tumours are rare tumours, accounting for around 1% of all digestive tumours [1]. They form a heterogeneous group of tumours with varying clinical characteristics, secretory and functional properties and evolution.

They are of epithelial origin and sometimes express specific markers known as neuroendocrine markers.

Most of these tumours are sporadic, but a genetic component has been reported in some cases [2].

The embryonic origin has long been suggested. In fact, the cells of the digestive tract derive from "pluripotential" cell progenitors, contrary to an old theory which held that these cells derived from the neural crest and then migrated to their final sites. This old theory has now been abandoned.

They can arise from any segment of the digestive tract, and can be differentiated or indifferentiated, secretory or non secretory, functional or non functional, and can even form part of syndromic associations such as multiple endocrine neoplasia type 1 (MEN1).

This anatomical and histopathological heterogeneity implies very broad therapeutic indications (symptomatic, curative, palliative treatment) and a highly variable prognosis depending on location, extension, histological type and whether or not the disease is secretory.

The aim of our retrospective study is to report the experience of the Gastroenterology Department of Nabeul in the management of gastroenteropancreatic neuroendocrine tumours, while specifying :

1)   The different epidemiological, clinical, therapeutic and prognostic aspects.

2)   Prognostic factors related to the terrain and the tumour itself, and by comparing our results with those published in the literature.

II METHODS

II.1. . Characteristics of the study :

This is a retrospective, cross-sectional study of 55 patients treated for gastroenteropancreatic neuroendocrine tumours in the gastroenterology and general surgery departments of Mohamed Taher Maamouri Hospital in Nabeul, over a 12-year period (January 2005 to December 2016).

Data were collected by consulting the medical records of patients in the gastroenterology and general surgery departments.

II.2. . Patients :

II .2.1. Inclusion criteria :

We included all patients with a digestive neuroendocrine tumour. The diagnosis was made clinically, biologically and radiologically. It was confirmed by histological and immunohistochemical examination of biopsies or the operative resection specimen.

II.2.2. Exclusion criteria :

All other histological types of tumour and non-digestive neuroendocrine tumours were excluded from the study.

II .2.3. Non-inclusion criteria :

We did not include in the study patients who were managed outside the study period and those in whom the diagnosis of NET was uncertain.

II.3. . Methods :

II.3.1.. Data collection :

As a source of data, we used :

- Medical records for patients treated on an outpatient or inpatient basis.
- Pathology reports from the general surgery department for patients undergoing surgery.
- Radiological examination reports
- Digestive endoscopy reports.

An information sheet containing clinical and paraclinical data was drawn up for each patient (Appendix 1).

II.3.2.. Anatomopathological study :

• The macroscopic appearance of the tumours was assessed either endoscopically or on surgical resection specimens. The size, colour and shape of the tumours were specified. Histological diagnosis was made on biopsies in 15 cases and on surgical specimens in 44 cases.

The following parameters have been specified:

• The degree of differentiation

• Mitotic index

• Vascular emboli and perineural sheathing

• Immunohistochemical data: general neuroendocrine markers (Chromogranin, Synaptophysin, etc.) and Ki67 were specified.

• Biopsies were taken during endoscopic examination for gastric, duodenal and recto-colonic sites, and under radiological guidance for hepatic sites.

II.3.3.. Histological grade and tumour stage :

The 55 digestive NETs in our series were classified according to WHO grade 2010 and UICC/AJCC Staging 7eme edition (Appendices 2, 3 and 4).

II.3.4.. Statistical analysis :

- Statistical data were entered and analysed using SPSS software (Statistical Package for the Social Sciences) version 22.0. The results were expressed as means, medians and

standard deviations for quantitative variables and as frequencies and percentages for qualitative variables.
-    In all statistical tests, the significance level was set at 0.05.

III RESULTS

II.4. 1. Epidemiological study :

II.4.1.1. Frequency and location :

Our study included 55 cases of digestive neuroendocrine tumours, i.e. 1.6% of all digestive tumours diagnosed in the gastroenterology and general surgery departments of the Med Taher Maamouri Hospital in Nabeul, between January 2005 and December 2016, a period of 12 years. They were distributed according to location as follows:

The appendix predominated in 41.8% of cases (n=23), followed by the pancreas in 14.5% (n=8). Figure 1 illustrates the distribution of the different digestive neuroendocrine tumours (NETs) according to tumour location.

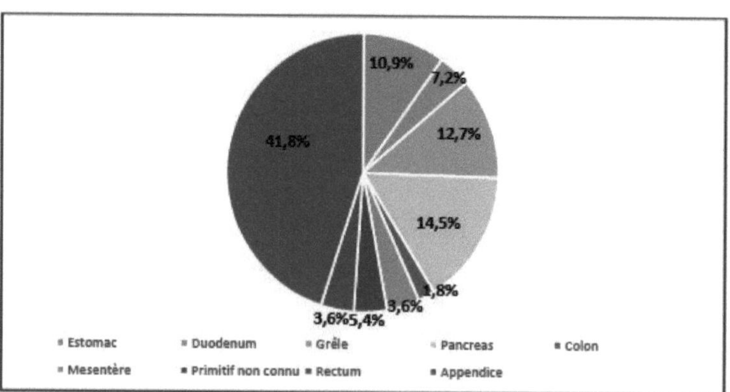

Figure 1: Distribution according to tumour location

II.4.2.2. Age distribution :

The average age of our patients was 43.3 years, with extremes of 11 and 80 years. Table I shows the age distribution of our patients according to tumour site.

Table I: Average age according to tumour site

Seat	Number of cases	Average age
Stomach	6	55,2
Duodenum	3	62
Grele	6	63
Pancreas	8	55
Appendix	23	26,8
Colon	1	76
Rectum	2	49
Mesentere	2	37,5
Grele + Mesentere	1	56
Primitive unknown	3	57
Total	55	43,3

Figure 2 shows the distribution of our patients by age group.

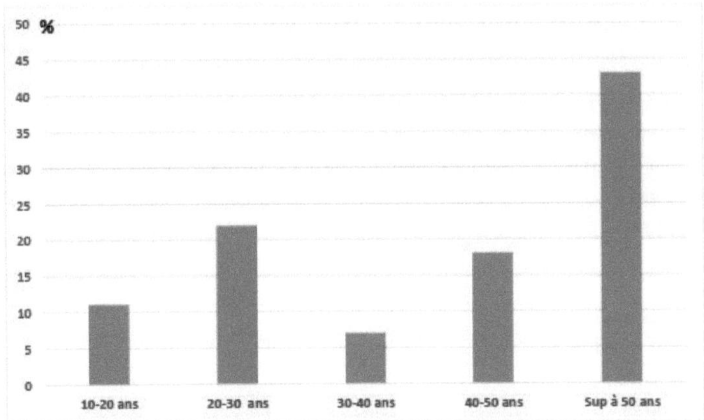

Figure 2: Breakdown of patients by age group

II.4.3.3. Breakdown by gender :

There was a slight female predominance, with 29 women (52.7%) and 26 men (47.3%), giving a sex ratio of 0.85. Table II shows the sex ratio by tumour site.

Table II: Breakdown of sex ratio by headquarters

Seat	Number	Men	Woman	Sex Ratio
Stomach	6	1	5	0,2
Duodenum	3	2	1	2
Grele	6	2	4	0.5
Pancreas	8	4	4	1
Appendix	23	10	13	0,76
Colon	1	1	0	-
Rectum	2	1	1	1
Mesentere	2	1	1	1
Primitive unknown	3	3	0	-
Grele + Mesentere	1	1	0	-
Total	55	26	29	0,89

111.2. Clinical study :

111.2.1. Patient history and habits:

Ш.2.1.1. Family background :

Our patients had no family history of cancer or NEM1.

111.2.1.2. Personal history:

Fifteen patients (27.2%) had a medical history: 3 were being monitored for diabetes and hypertension, 4 were diabetic, 3 were hypertensive, 2 were dyslipidemic, and 3 patients with gastric NET had unrecognised atrophic gastritis.

Two patients had undergone surgery for a stenosing ulcer and had had a GEA (Gastro-entero anastomosis).

111.2.1.3. Habits :

Nine patients (16.3%) were smokers and 3 (5.4%) were chronic alcoholics.

111.2.1.4. Circumstances of discovery :

The mean duration of symptomatology was 5.4 months, ranging from 3 days to 18 months.

Abdominal pain was the main symptom, occurring in 43 cases (78.1%). A typical appendicular syndrome was indicative of appendicular NET in 22 cases (40%). The different circumstances of discovery are summarised in Table III. Table IV illustrates the circumstances of discovery according to site.

Table III: Circumstances of discovery

Circumstances of discovery	Number	%
Abdominal pain	43	78,1
Change in general condition	6	10,9
Chest pain	3	5,4
Vomiting	3	5,4
Recurrent hypoglycemia	1	1,8
Sub-occlusive syndrome	4	7,2
Rectal syndrome	1	1,8
Abdominal mass	2	3,6
Flush syndrome	2	3,6

Table IV: Circumstances of discovery by location

Location	Clinical/biological signs/ syndromes
Stomach	Abdominal pain: 80%. Digestive haemorrhage: 20%. Alteration of general condition (AEG): 40 Anemia: 20%.
Duodenum	Abdominal pain + General improvement: 100%. Vomiting: 60%.
Grele	Abdominal pain: 66 Diarrhoea: 16 Change in general condition: 16 Occlusive syndrome: 33 Incidental diagnosis (Per-operative): 16%.
Appendix	Abdominal pain: 100%. Fever: 43 Carcinoid syndrome: 1.8% (1 case)
Colon/Rectum	Occlusive syndrome: 33 Chest pain: 33 Anal pain: 33 Change in general condition: 66
Pancreas	Abdominal pain: 100%. Alteration of general condition: 75%. Vomiting: 14 Epigastric mass: 25%.
Mesentere	Abdominal pain: 100%. Occlusive syndrome: 50%.

Image 1 shows erythrosis of the face and hands as part of a flush syndrome in a patient with a secondary hepatic NET of unknown origin.

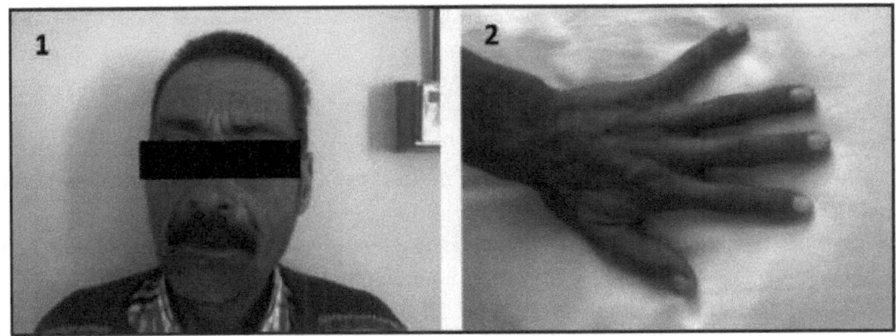

Image 1 and 2: Erythrosis of the face and hands

111.4.　　Paraclinical examinations :
111.4.1.　　Endoscopic examinations :
111.4.1.1.　Oeso-gastro-duodenal endoscopy:
Twenty-three patients underwent oeso-gastro-duodenal endoscopy (EOGD). It revealed the tumour in 9 cases: 6 cases of gastric NET, one case of bulbar NET and two cases of ampullary NET.

- 　+ The endoscopic appearance of gastric NETs was:
- 　A polypoid ulcerated fundic formation measuring 8 mm in 2 cases.
- 　Atrophic fundic gastritis with multiple ulcerated polyploid formations in 2 cases.
- 　Multiple resophageal, gastric and bulbar ulcerations in one case.
- 　An ulcerated budding formation in one case.
- 　> For bulbar NET: Two millimetric bulbar polyploid formations.

- 　For the two ampullary locations: duodenoscopy in one case revealed a swollen ampulla of Vater with no visible tumour proliferation. The diagnosis was subsequently confirmed by echoendoscopy. In the 2eme case, EOGD showed a congestive and ulcerated swollen ampulla.

111.4.1.2.　Colonoscopy :
It was carried out in 14 patients (25.4%) and revealed tumours in 4 cases (7.2%): 1 in the colon, at the level of the caecal fundus, with an ulcerating-bourging appearance, 2 in the middle rectum, in the form of a sessile polyp in one case and a submucosal formation in the other, and 1 in the last loop of the ileum, with a polypoid appearance.

111.4.2.　　Imaging :
111.4.2.1.　Abdominal ultrasound :
It was carried out in 28 patients (51%); it was normal in 9 cases (16.3%) and had identified the tumour in 19 cases (34.5%). It concluded :

- 　Multinodular liver with a secondary appearance in 6 cases: 1 case of pancreatic tumour, 3 cases of unknown origin, 1 case of grafted NET with hepatic metastases and one case of metachronous recurrence in the liver of a rectal NET.
- 　Two cases of pancreatic NET: in one patient, abdominal ultrasound revealed a heterogeneous hypoechogenic right flank lateral wall mass 11x30 mm in diameter. In 2eme cases, a left inter-spleno-renal retro-peritoneal tissue mass was found.
- 　A case of jejunal NET: abdominal ultrasound showed a left flank mass 42x38 mm in diameter, 68 mm high, with a hypoechoic wall, 13 mm thick and cocardized on axial sections.
- 　Two cases of mesenteric NET in which the tumour was described on ultrasound as a

voluminous cystic mass in the first case, and large coeliomesenteric adenopathies in the second.

- In the case of gastrinoma, ultrasound showed a nodule in the back cavity of the epiplons, which was hypoechogenic, regular and 2 cm in diameter.

- Six cases of appendiceal NETs where abdominal ultrasound showed minimal right iliac fossa effusion or signs of acute appendicitis in the context of exploration for an appendicular syndrome.

- A case of colonic NET in which ultrasound revealed a tumour mass in the right flank, probably in the colon, confirmed by computed tomography (CT) and colonoscopy.

111.4.2.2. Thoracic-abdominal-pehrial CT scan:

It was carried out in 32 patients (58.1%); it was abnormal in 28 cases (50.9%).

It objectified the primary tumour in 21 cases (38.1%):

<u>+ Six cases of NET of the gallbladder:</u>

- Stenosis of the last loop of the eye

- Nodular tissue thickening in the jejunal lumen and left flank enhanced by contrast medium.

- Intraperitoneal tissue formation in a patient with a double location in the gallbladder and mesentery.

- A frozen loop with no parietal enhancement and a "feces sign" suggestive primarily of mesenteric infarction.

- Circumferential thickening of the walls of the terminal ileum, creating a pseudo-mass measuring 35 mm, with another ileal parietal mass at a distance, suggesting a 2eme location.

- Colonic dilatation with disparity in calibre between the graft intestine and the right colon and a secondary multinodular liver.

Image 3 (A and B) illustrates the scannographic appearance of a grafted NET.

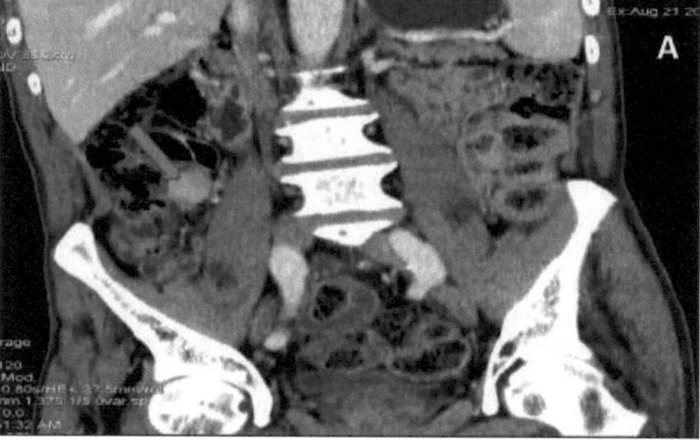

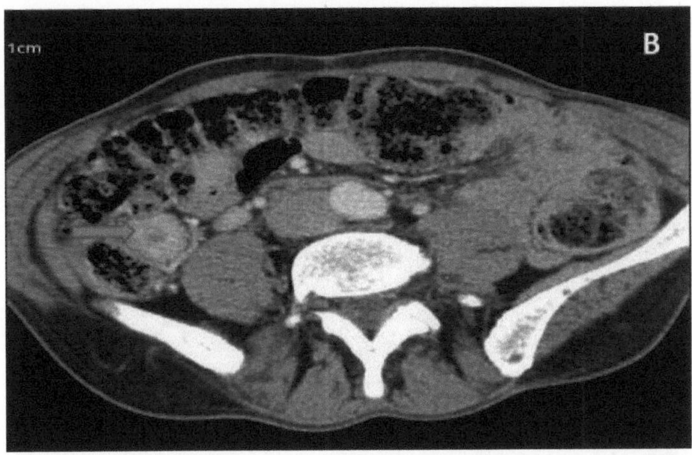

Image 3: Abdominal CT scan A: coronal section. B: axial section at portal time Greclic NET (arrows) in a 57-year-old man.

^ A case of gastric NET: regular and moderate thickening of the wall of the gastric antrum extended to the lesser curvature with integrity of the perigastric fat.

■+ Eight cases of pancreatic NET:

- An isodense tissue mass in the tail of the pancreas.
- An inter-splenopancreatic tissue mass, probably of pancreatic origin.
- Thickening of the posterior retrohepatic wall in contact with the posterior pillar of the diaphragm. Additional MRI confirmed pancreatic origin.
- A cephalic pancreatic mass 60x50 mm in diameter in contact with the portal trunk.
- An infiltrating mass in the tail of the pancreas with hepatic, lymph node and vascular extension.
- Tissue ganglion magma opposite the head of the pancreas.
- Two cases of tissue thickening opposite the head of the pancreas.

Images 4, 5 and 6 show CT scans of 3 pancreatic NETs.

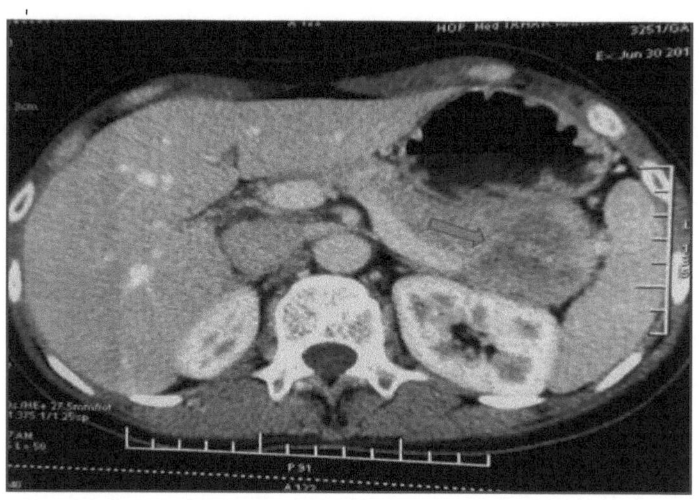

Image 4: Abdominal CT scan (axial section at pancreatic time) showing a pancreatic NET
revealed by abdominal pain in a 34-year-old patient
(arrow).

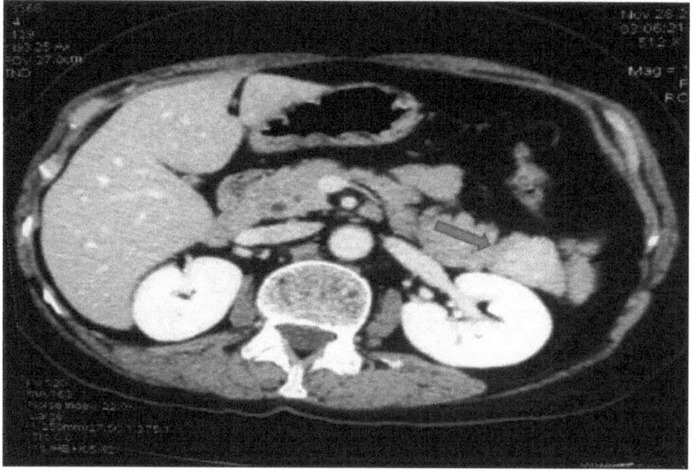

Image 5: Abdominal CT scan (axial section at arterial time) showing a pancreatic NET
(arrow) in a 62-year-old patient.

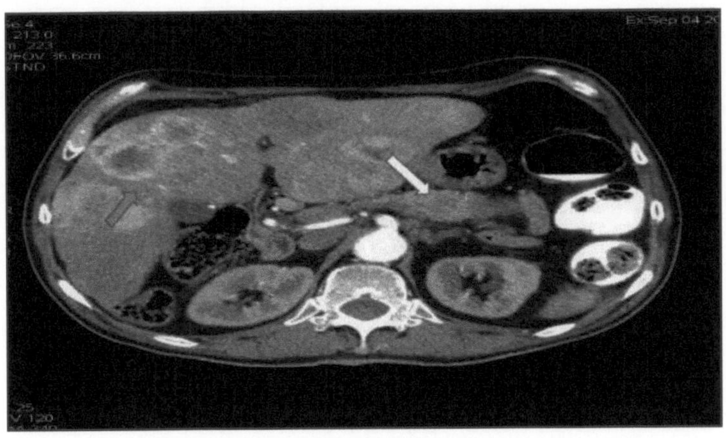

Image 6: Abdominal CT scan (axial section at arterial time) illustrating a pancreatic tail NET
(white arrow) with hepatic metastases (blue arrow) in a
66-year-old
patient.

-> <u>Two mesenteric tumours:</u>

- An intraperitoneal cystic mass with multiple compartments and haemorrhagic content.

- Two intraperitoneal masses, one of which depends on the digestive wall and develops exoluminally.

^ <u>Two duodenal tumours (ampullary):</u>

In the 1er case: significant dilatation of the main bile duct and intrahepatic bile ducts with no visible obstruction. Echoendoscopy confirmed an ampullary tumour. In the 2eme cases: regular hypodense thickening opposite the pancreatic head.

<u>A colonic tumour:</u> heterogeneous mass in the right iliac fossa, 85 mm in diameter, protruding into the cecal lumen.

<u>A rectal tumour: a</u> tissue mass in the left lateral wall of the upper rectum.

CT scans **showed hepatic metastases** in 7 cases:

-> Three cases in which the primary tumour remained unknown with a multinodular liver on ultrasound and CT scan.

+ Two cases of NET of the graft, one of which was discovered incidentally per-operatively during exploration of two hepatic nodules for which percutaneous biopsy was inconclusive on 2 occasions. In the 2eme cases, CT scans showed two nodules in segments 5 and 7 with heterogeneous enhancement at arterial time, associated with two contiguous mesenteric tissue masses suggestive of adenopathy.

+ A case of NET of the tail of the pancreas.

+ A case of rectal NET resected endoscopically and subsequently treated surgically (anterior resection) with metastatic recurrence in the liver after 4 years.

Images 7, 8 and 9 show scans of liver metastases in 3 patients.

Neuroendocrine origin was suggested on CT scan in 7 cases: 2 hepatic metastases, one of unknown origin and the other secondary to a pancreatic NET, one colonic NET, 3 pancreatic NETs and one gallbladder NET.

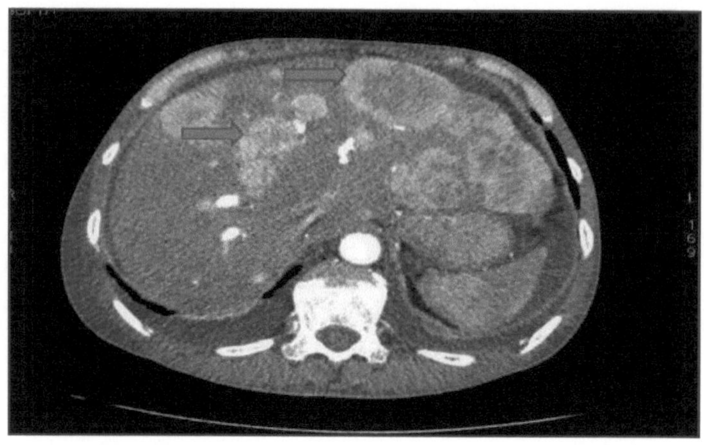

Image 7: Abdominal CT scan (axial section at arterial time) showing hepatic metastases (arrows) from a NET of unknown origin.

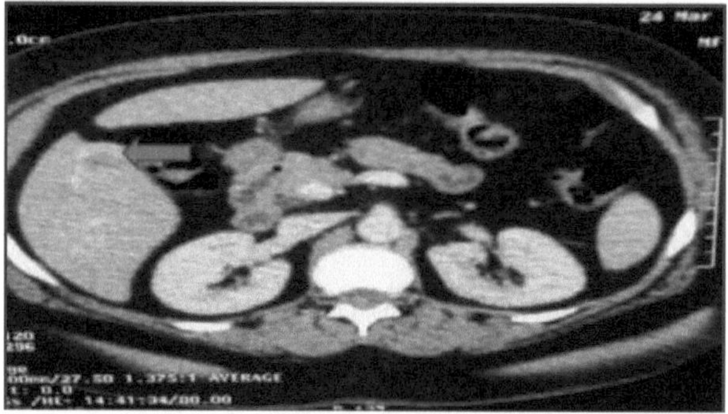

Image 8: Abdominal CT scan (portal axial slice) showing a hepatic metastasis
of a NET of the graft (arrow).

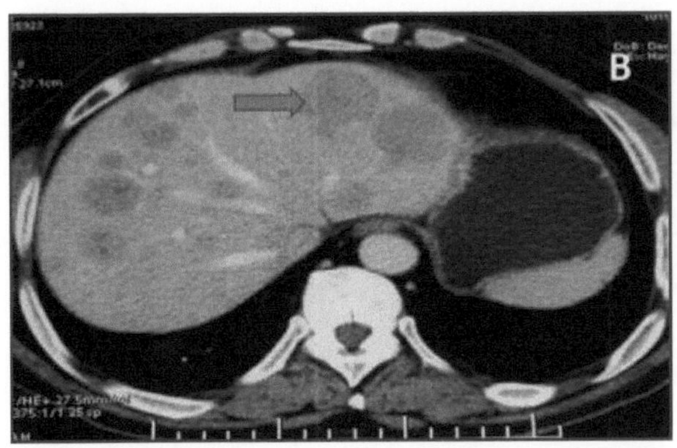

Image 9: Abdominal CT scan (axial sections A+B at portal time) showing multiple hepatic metastases (arrows) in a patient operated on for a mesenteric NET, which had progressed after 6 years in the form of hepatic localisations.

111.4.2.3.   Octreoscanner®:

It was performed in only 17 patients (30.9%). No patient with appendiceal involvement underwent octreoscan, as post-operative surveillance is not indicated for appendiceal NETs < 2 cm that have been completely resected (R0), without lymph node metastases or vascular invasion. OCT revealed distant localisations in 4 patients (7.2%). The results of octreoscans in four patients are detailed in Table V and the images in Figures 10 and 11.

Table V: Results of pathological octreoscans

Patient	Location of the primary tumour	Octreoscanner
Patient 1	Hepatic metastases of unknown origin	Octreotide-binding left jugulocarotid lymph node discharge suggestive of NE origin
Patient 2	Hepatic metastases of unknown origin	Hepatic nodules expressing somatostatin receptors
Patient 3	Pancreas head	Large area of intense, multifocal hyperfixation involving the epigastric region.
Patient 4	Hepatic metastases of unknown origin	Hepatic nodules expressing somatostatin receptors

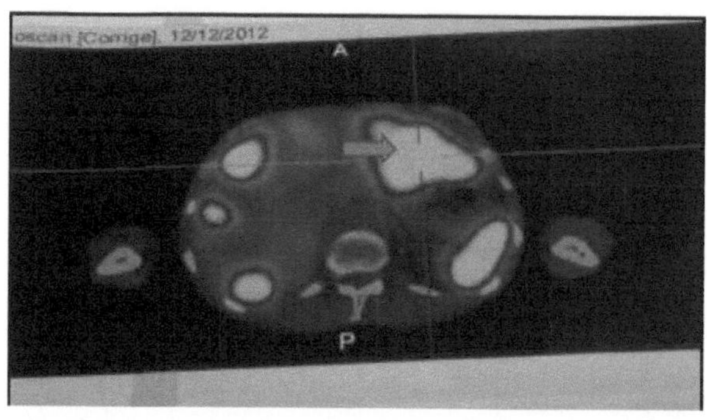

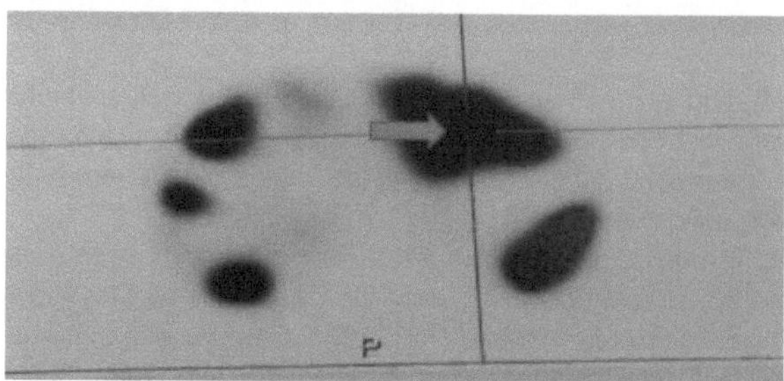

Image 10: Octreoscan images showing
hepatic nodules
strongly expressing somatostatin receptors
(arrows), arguing for their endocrine origin.

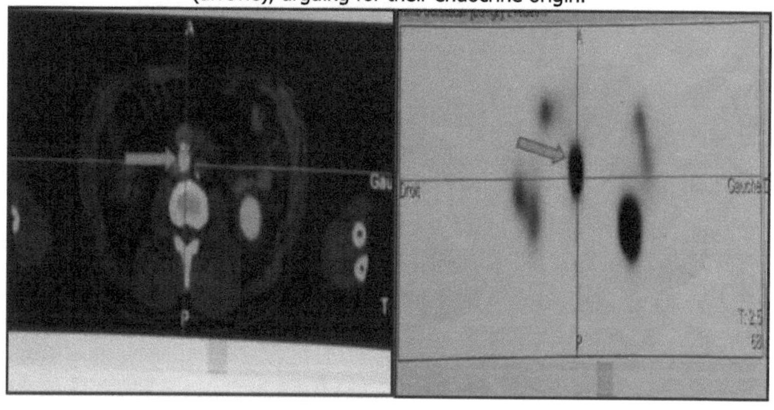

Image 11 : Octreoscan films showing intense hyperfixation
in the epigastric region (arrow), in relation to an inter-aortic-caval metastasis
of a pancreatic NET.

111.4.2.4. *Magnetic resonance imaging :*

Abdominal magnetic resonance imaging (MRI) was performed in 3 patients (5.4%):
-    Two patients with pancreatic NET:

In one patient, pancreatic MRI revealed multiple compressive pancreatic nodular lesions over the head of the pancreas, varying in size, the two largest measuring 47 x 36 mm and 47 x 26 mm in diameter respectively. They compressed the duodenal bulb, the 2eme and the 3eme portion of the duodenum.

In the 2eme patient, pancreatic MRI showed a round heterogeneous lesion with T1 hyposignal and T2 hypersignal measuring 30 x 25 mm in diameter.

- A case of hepatic metastases of a grafted NET: MRI showed 2 well-bounded, rounded hepatic nodules in segments V and VII measuring 28 x 25 mm and 23 x 20 mm in diameter with T1 hyposignal and T2 hypersignal, which were homogeneously intensely enhanced from arterial time without wash-out.

Image 12 illustrates the MRI appearance of hepatic neuroendocrine metastases from a gracilic primary.

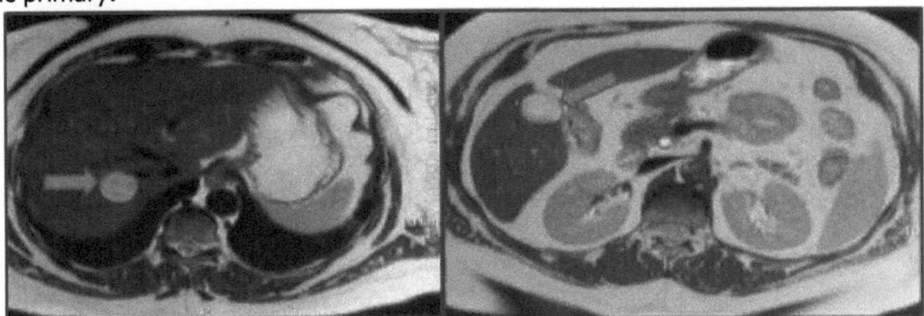

Image 12 : Hepatic MRI (2 axial slices in T2-weighted sequence) showing hepatic metastases (arrows) from an NET of the graft revealed by a multinodular liver.

111.5. Biological tests and electrocardiogram :

111.5.1. Chromogranin 'A' and 5 urinary HIAA :

Five patients had a chromogranin A blood test. It was elevated (>100 ng/mL) in 4 cases and normal in one.

One patient had a urinary 5 HIAA assay, which showed a value of 1818 jmol/L (normal value less than 47 |jmol/24h).

111.5.2. Glycemia :

Blood glucose levels on admission were normal in all our patients.

111.5.3. Electrocardiogram :

The electrocardiogram, performed in 15 patients (27.2%), was normal in all cases.

111.6. Anatomopathological examination :

111.6.1. Type of sample :

111.6.1.1. Biopsy :

The diagnosis of NET was made on the basis of biopsy data in 15 cases (27.2%):

- Six cases of gastric NET
- Two cases of duodenal NET: 1 patient had 2 bulbar millimetre polypoid formations and 2eme had an ampulla of Vater suspected of degeneration at endoscopy confirmed by biopsy data.
- Four cases of NET with hepatic metastases: 1 case of pancreatic NET metastatic to the liver and 3 cases of hepatic metastases of unknown origin.
- Two cases of rectal NET and 1 case of colonic NET.

Ш.6.1.2. Piece operator :

The diagnosis was made in the operating theatre in 44 cases (80%):

- Twenty-three cases of appendiceal NETs, operated on as part of an appendicular

syndrome.
- Seven cases of pancreatic NETs
- Seven cases of NET of the gallbladder were reported, one of which had a dual location in the gallbladder and mesentery.
- Two cases of mesenteric NETs
- A case of colonic NET.
- Two cases of rectal NET.
- Two cases of ampullary NET in a piece of cephalic duodeno-pancreatectomy (CPD).

### 111.6.2.	Macroscopy :

Tumour size ranged from 2 mm to 70 mm, with a mean of 19.65 mm.

The gastric NETs were polypoid in appearance, associated with atrophic fundic gastritis in 3 cases, and had a budding and ulcerated appearance in one case.

Duodenal NETs presented in 2 different forms: a bulbar NET in the form of polypoid millimetric formations and an ulcerated blister for the two ampullary NETs.

The colonic NET had a budding and ulcerated appearance on endoscopy.

The two rectal NETs had the appearance of a non-ulcerated submucosal formation in one patient, and the form of a sessile polyp in the other 2 .[eme]

Table VI summarises tumour size according to location.

Table VI: Average tumour size by location

Location	Number	Max size (mm)	Minimum size (mm)	Average size (mm)
Stomach	6	14	2	8
Duodenum	3	40	5	22,5
Grele	6	40	15	26,6
Appendix	23	70	2	8,91
Colon	1	-	-	-
Rectum	2	53	12	32,5
Pancreas	8	60	6	37
Mesentere	2	60	27	43,5
Primitive unknown	3	-	-	-
Grele + mesentere	1	-	-	-

Figure 3 shows the distribution of patients according to tumour size.

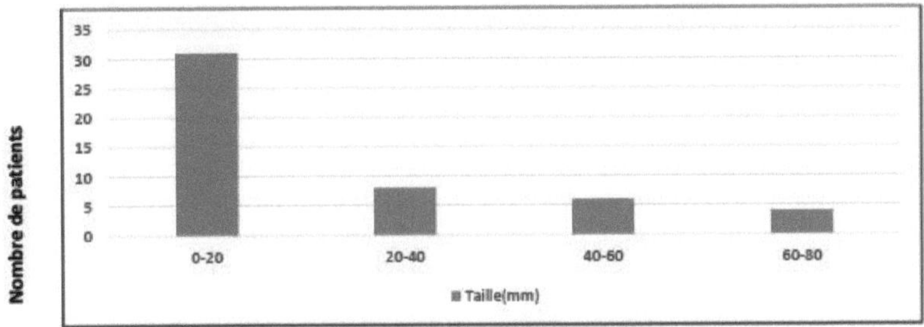

Figure 3: Distribution of patients by tumour size

111.6.3.   Microscopy :

111.6.3.1.   Tumour differentiation :

6.3.1.1.   Well differentiated NETs:

In 53 cases (96%), tumour proliferation was well differentiated. The tumours were gastric (6 cases), gallbladder (6 cases), appendicular (23 cases), pancreatic (8 cases), mesenteric (2 cases), rectal (2 cases), duodenal (2 cases) and 4 hepatic sites of unknown origin.

6.3.1.2.   Not very differentiated NETs:

Tumour proliferation was only slightly different in 2 cases: one case of colonic NET and one case of grafted NET. In both cases, the tumours were large-cell.

111.   6.3.2 Mitotic index :

The mitotic index was accurate in 39 cases (71%), ranging from 0 to 27 mitoses per 10 fields at high magnification, with an average of 3 mitoses.

111.6.4.   Immunohistochemistry :

111.6.4.1.   Differentiation markers :

- **Chromogranin A :**

It was tested in all cases, with a positive result in 80% of cases. Marking was weak in 2 cases.

- **Synaptophysin :**

It was tested in 40 cases (72.7%), with a positive result in 68.6% of cases.

- **CD56 :**

It was positive in 10 cases (18.1%). Half of these patients were negatively labelled for chromogranin A.

- **CK 7 :**

Positive labelling for CK7 was observed in 8 cases (14.5%).

Figure 4 illustrates the rate of positivity of the different differentiation markers in our patients.

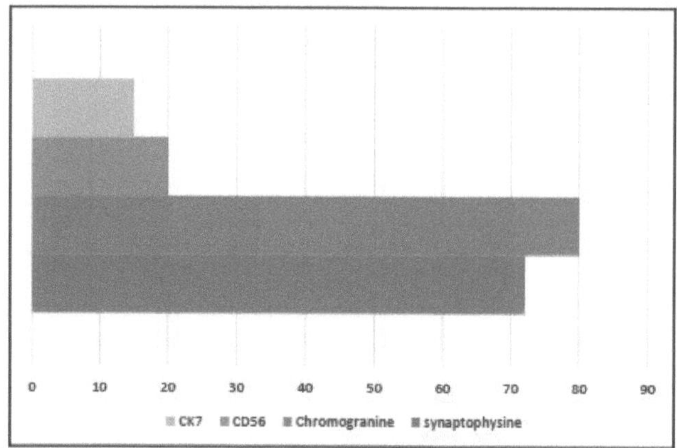

Figure 4: Positive rate of tumour differentiation markers

Image 13 illustrates the histological appearance of a greclic NET with intense labelling by synaptophysin and chromogranin.

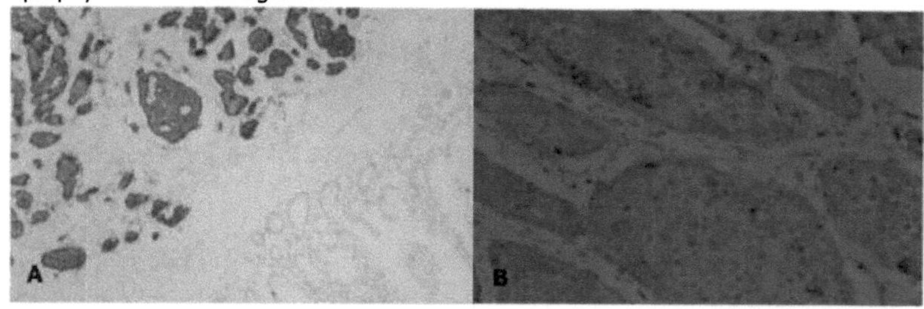

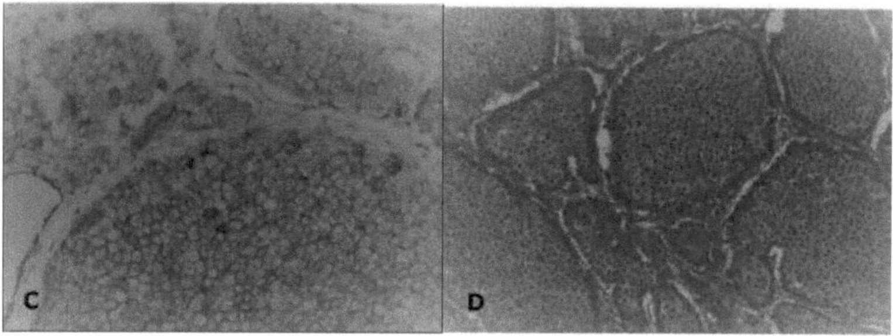

Image 13: NET of the grele

A: Intense expression of Chromogranin

B: Synaptophysin immunohistochemical labelling

C: CD56 membrane expression

D : Tracheal appearance/richly vascularised NET

1.1.1.2.   2. Proliferation index (Ki67) :

It was carried out in all cases. It varied between 0 and 40%, with an average of 5%. It was greater than or equal to 20% in 6 cases. Table VII shows the distribution of mean Ki67 according to tumour location. Figure 5 shows the Ki67 profile.

Table VII: Average Ki67 by tumour site

Location	Number	Average Ki67(%)
Appendix	23	1,08
Colon	1	20
Rectum	2	3
Pancreas	8	8
Stomach	6	5,2
Duodenum	3	11,5
Grele	6	10,3
Mesentere	2	2
Primitive unknown	3	21,5
Grele + mesentere	1	1

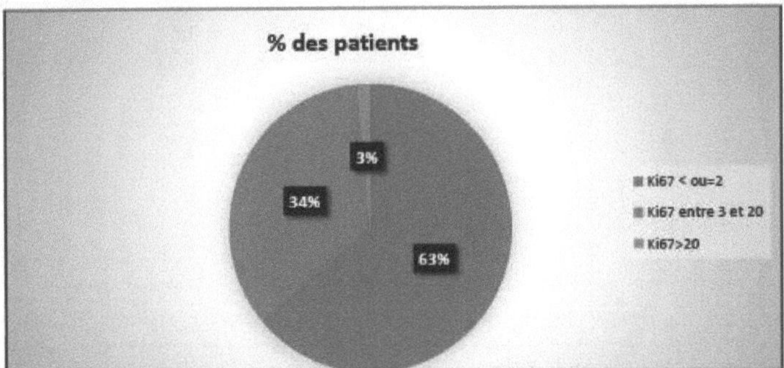

Figure 5: ki67 profile

111.6.5. Histological grade according to ENETS :

According to the histological grade, we were able to classify the tumours as follows:

- Grade 1: 30 cases (54.5%)

- Grade 2: 21 cases (38.1%)

- Grade 3: 2 cases (3.6%)

The remaining two cases were mixed NETs.

111.6.6. WHO 2010 classification and tumour stage :

111.6.6.1. WHO 2010:

According to the WHO 2010 classification, our patients were divided into :

- TNE G1: 30 cases (54.5%)

- TNE G2: 21 cases (38.1%)

- Neuroendocrine carcinoma: 2 cases (3.6%)

- Mixed adeno-neuroendocrine carcinoma: 2 cases (3.6%)

111.6.6.2. Dynamic stage (UICC/AJCC 7th edition):

The tumours were classified according to AJCC 7eme edition as follows:

- Stage 0 (tumour in situ of the stomach): 1 case (1.8%)

23

- Stage I: 31 cases (56.3%)

- Stage IIA: 9 cases (16.3%)

- Stage IIB: 2 cases (3.6%)

- Stage IIIA: 1 case (1.8%)

- Stage IIIB: 2 cases (3.6%)

- Stage IV: 4 cases (7.2%)

- Unclassifiable tumour: 5 cases (9%)

Figure 6 shows the distribution of different tumour stages according to tumour site.

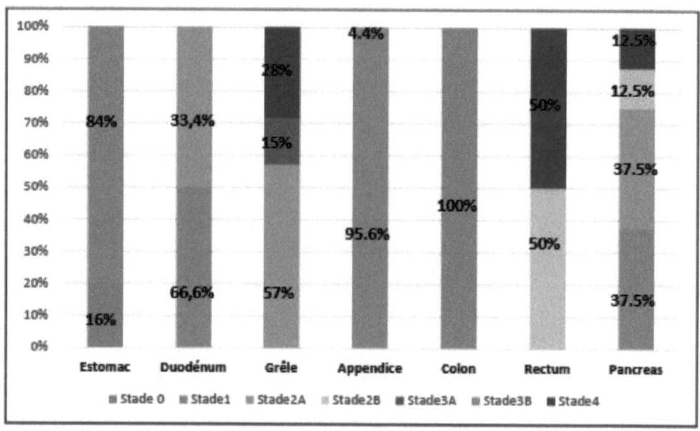

Figure 6. Distribution of tumour stages by site

III.7. Extension assessment :

- Thoraco-abdomino-pelvic TDM was performed in 32 cases (58.1%), with distant metastases identified in 10 cases (18.1%):
Hepatic metastases in 7 cases (12.7%).
Node metastases in 3 cases (5.4%).

- An octreoscan was performed in 16 cases (29%), revealing distant localisations in 3 cases (5.4%).

Table VIII summarises the different locations of primary tumours and the site of metastases on CT and CT octreoscan.

Table VIII. Location of metastases

Patient no.	Original location	CT SCAN	Octreoscanner®
Patient 1	Unknown	Multinodular liver	Left jugulo-carotid lymph node discharge fixing octreotide suggestive of NE origin
Patient 2	Unknown	Multinodular liver	Hepatic nodules expressing somatostatin receptors

Patient 3	Unknown	Multinodular liver	-
Patient 4	Grele	Multinodular liver	-
Patient 5	Grele	Multinodular liver	-
Patient 6	Colon	Metastasis of lymph nodes	-
Patient 7	Pancreas head	Metastasis of lymph nodes	Wide range of intense, multifocal hyperfixation involving the epigastric region
Patient 8	Pancreas tail	Multinodular liver	-
Patient 9	Mesentere	Metastasis of lymph nodes	-
Patient 10	Rectum	Multinodular liver	

(NE: Neuroendocrine)

III.8. Therapeutic management :

III.8.1. Medical treatment :

Medical treatment was initiated in 15 patients (27.2%).

III.8.1.1 Proton pump inhibitors (PPIs):

They were used in 3 patients:

J A patient with a gastrinoma

J A patient with gastric NET in atrophic gastritis.

J A patient with a mesenteric NET with an anastomotic ulcer on an AEG.

111.8.1.2.   Somatostatin analogues :

They were prescribed for 6 patients (10.9%):

J Three patients with hepatic metastases of an unknown neuroendocrine primary.

J A patient with a pancreatic head NET with lymph node metastases. Analogues were started after CPP.

J A patient with a pancreatic NET with hepatic metastases.

J A patient with a NET of the graft with hepatic metastases. Treatment was initiated after surgical resection of the primary tumour.

111.8.1.3.   Chemotherapy :

It was indicated in six patients (10.9%):

-   A patient with a pancreatic TUMOUR with hepatic metastases underwent palliative chemotherapy after progressing on somatostatin analogues.

-   A case of mid-rectal TNE initially treated endoscopically (polypectomy), then with additional anterior resection due to incomplete endoscopic exeresis. Chemotherapy was prescribed for recurrence in the form of hepatic metastases after 48 months of remission.

-   A patient with a NET of the graft with hepatic metastases. The graft tumour was resected and the patient underwent post-operative chemotherapy.

-   A patient operated for a mesenteric NET with progression to hepatic localisations after 72 months of evolution.

-   emeTwo patients with mixed adeno-neuroendocrine carcinoma: one with an ampullary location who underwent DPC and received adjuvant Gemcitabine, and one with a gastric siege who underwent sub-total gastrectomy with surgical tumour border and presence of perineural sheathing, indicating adjuvant chemotherapy with Folfox (Oxaliplatin + Folinic acid and 5-fluorouracil).

111.8.2. Surgical treatment :

Surgical treatment was performed in 44 cases (80%).

Surgery was curative in 37 cases (67.2%) and non-carcinological in the remaining 7 cases; 2 patients with NET of the graft with hepatic metastases underwent graft resection, and four patients with lymph node metastases underwent surgery on the primary tumour. One patient had undergone subtotal gastrectomy for a mixed adeno-neuroendocrine gastric carcinoma with a surgical tumour boundary on pathological examination.

All patients who underwent surgery were distributed as follows:

- Twenty-three patients (41.8%) had appendectomy alone and the surgical margins were healthy.

- A patient with a right colonic TUMOUR underwent right hemi-colectomy.

- Four patients had a DPC: two patients had an ampullary TUMOUR and two had a pancreatic head NET.

- Tumour resection was performed in 9 cases (16.3%): two cases of primary mesenteric NET, one of which was a gastrinoma, 1 case of graft NET associated with a mesenteric site, and 6 cases of graft NET.

- Left pancreatectomy was performed in 4 cases.

- Anterior rectal resection for middle rectal NET was performed in 2 cases.

- Subtotal gastrectomy for a mixed adeno-neuroendocrine gastric tumour in one case.

Figure 7 illustrates the different surgical procedures performed on our patients.

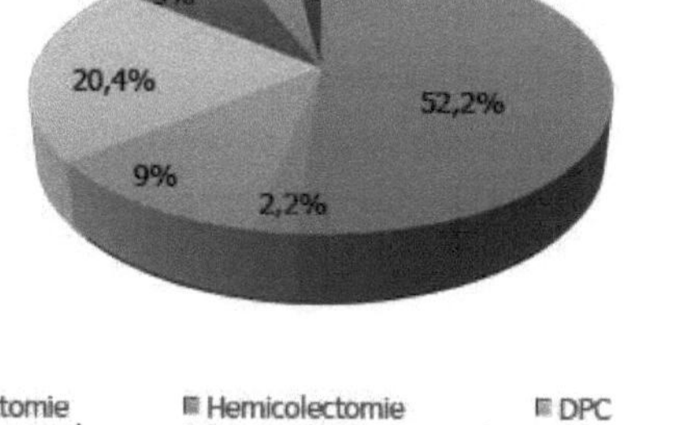

Figure 7: Different surgical procedures performed on our patients

111.8.3. Endoscopic treatment :

Two patients had undergone polypectomy.

One patient had ulcerated polypoid formations, 8 mm in diameter, on endoscopic atrophic fundic gastritis, which anatomopathological examination confirmed to be neuroendocrine. The exeresis was complete.

The 2eme case was a tumour of the middle rectum which appeared as a sessile polyp 12mm in diameter. The endoscopic examination was incomplete, indicating that further surgery was required.

Figure 8 illustrates the different therapeutic modalities in our patients.

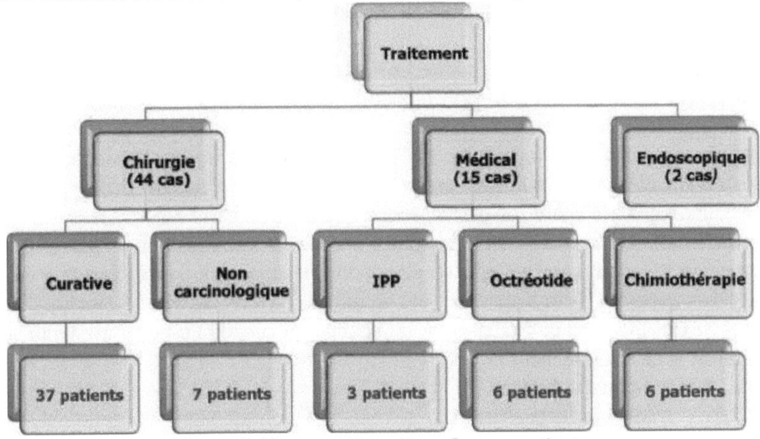

Figure 8: Therapeutic options for our patients

III.9. Survival, progression and prognostic factors :

111.9.1.   Average survival :

The mean survival time was 51 months, with extremes of 2 and 96 months. The table IX reports average survival rates according to location.

Table IX. Average survival by location

Location	Minimum survival time (months)	Maximum survival time (months)	Mean survival (months)
Stomach	38	96	62,8
Duodenum	12	26	19
Grele	2	48	20,7
Mesentere	36	48	42
Appendix	12	96	50,3
Colon	-	-	3
Rectum	12	48	30
Pancreas	2	36	11,6
Metastases from an unknown primary	3	4	3,5

111.9.2.   Evolution :

A patient operated for a colonic NET died after 3 months' follow-up.

Eighteen patients were lost to follow-up after an average of 28.2 months (extremes: 2 and 96 months).

The outcome was favourable in 32 cases (58%): 4 cases of gastric NET, 1 case of duodenal NET (ampullary), 5 cases of NET of the graft, 1 case of NET with dual graft and mesenteric localisation, 17 cases of appendicular NET, 3 cases of pancreatic NET and one case of primary mesenteric NET.

A patient with a pancreatic NET with hepatic metastases was initially treated with somatostatin analogues. Progression was marked by a progression of metastases under treatment, indicating that he should be put on chemotherapy.

Progression with chemotherapy was marked by tumour progression after a mean follow-up time of 11 months.

A patient underwent surgery for a rectal NET after incomplete endoscopic resection, and presented with recurrence in the form of hepatic metastases after 48 months. Systemic chemotherapy was indicated.

One patient, operated for a mesenteric NET, progressed to secondary hepatic localisations after 72 months of follow-up and was referred for palliative chemotherapy.

A patient undergoing surgery for gastric adeno-neuroendocrine carcinoma was started on adjuvant chemotherapy. A scan after 3 months showed progression in the form of hepatic metastases. A 2eme case of mixed adeno-neuroendocrine ampullary tumour was treated with adjuvant chemotherapy, with a scan showing no tumour recurrence after 12 months.

A case of NET of the head of the pancreas in a patient who had refused surgery with stable lesions on CT scan after 42 months.

111.9.3. Prognostic factors :

111.9.3.1. Histological grade :

WHO grade reduced survival. Indeed, 3-year survival for grade 1 was 100%, whereas it fell to 50% for grade 2. Figure 9 illustrates the survival curve according to WHO grade.

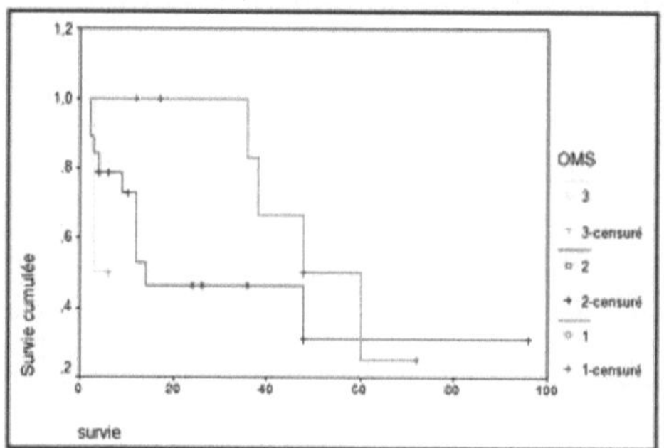

Figure 9: Survival curve according to WHO grade

111.9.3.2. Ki67 :

Survival at 1 year was better for a Ki67 of less than 10% (90% versus 62%), whereas it was reversed at 5 years: approximately 20% for a Ki67 of less than 10% versus 62% for a Ki67 > 10%, with no significant difference; this is probably due to other factors such as age and the presence of metastases. Figure 10 shows the survival curve according to Ki67 level.

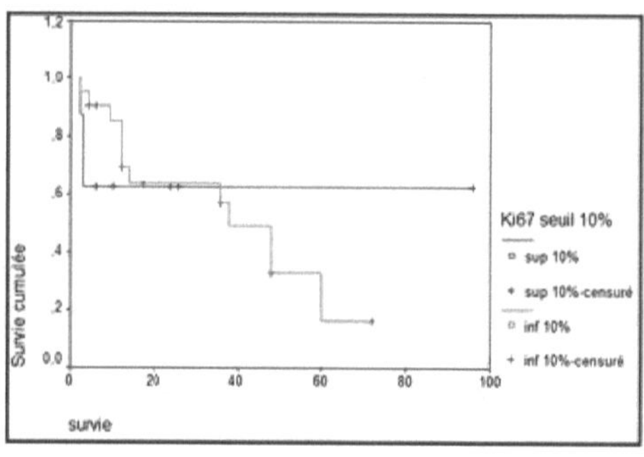

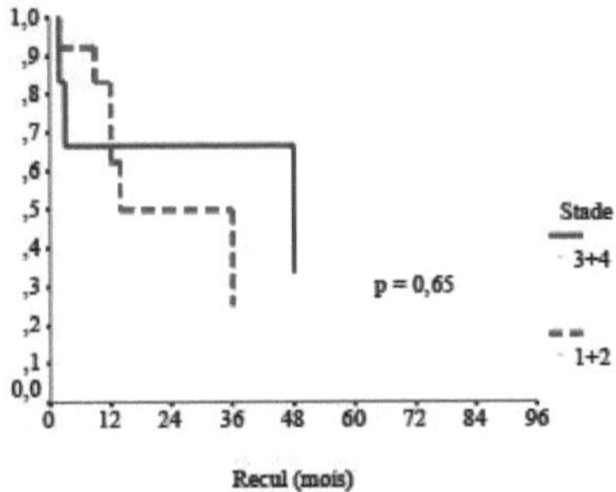

Figure 10: Survival curve according to Ki67 level

111.9.3.3. Tumour stage :

There was no significant difference in overall survival between the different tumour stages (p=0.65). Figure 11 shows the survival curve according to tumour stage.

Figure 11: Survival curve by tumour stage

111.9.3.4. Tumour cell :

Tumour size less than or equal to 30 mm was associated with better survival than tumour size > 30 mm (3-year survival = 80% versus 50%), with no significant difference. Figure 12 shows the survival curve according to tumour size.

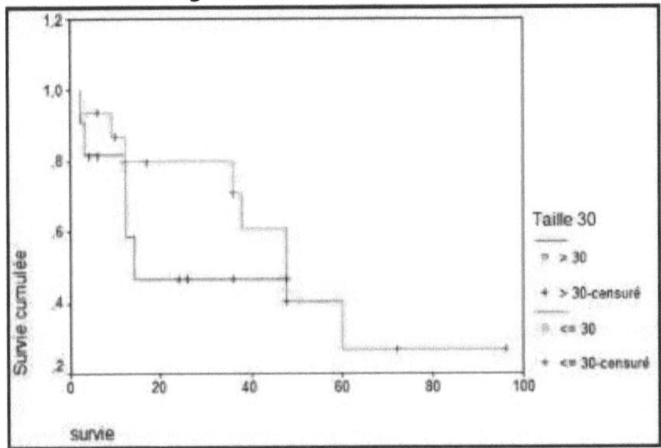

Figure 12: Survival curve according to tumour size

III. 9.3.5. Degree of differentiation :

We found significantly better survival in patients with well-differentiated NET compared with those with non-differentiated NET. Figure 13 shows the survival curve according to the degree of tumour differentiation.

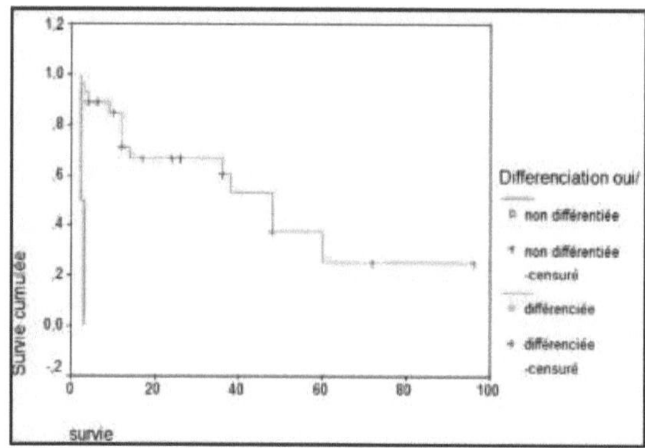

Figure 13: Survival curve according to tumour differentiation

III. 9.3.6. Tumour site :

Tumour location significantly reduced overall survival in our patients. Survival at 3 years was 90% for the graft and mesentery compared with 25% for the pancreas (p=0.0078). Figure 14 shows the survival curve according to tumour location.

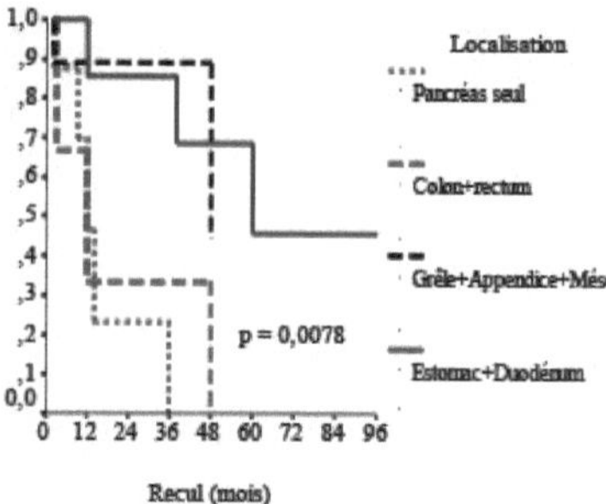

Figure 14: Survival curve by tumour site

Ш.9.3.7. Metastases and survival :

The presence of lymph node metastases and distant metastases reduced survival. Survival at 3 years without metastases was 65% compared with 55% in the presence of metastases. At 5 years, metastasis-free survival was 50% compared with almost zero survival in the presence of metastases. Figure 15 shows the survival curve according to the presence or absence of metastases.

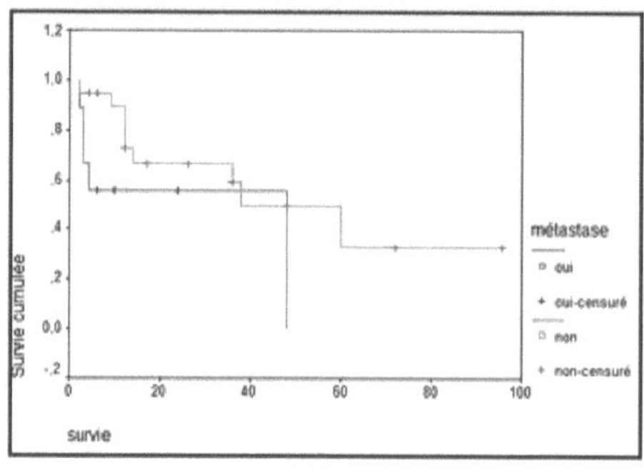

Figure 15: Survival curve by metastasis

111.10. Study of correlations :

111.10.1. Histological grade and histopronostic parameters :

Histological grade was significantly correlated with tumour size (p=0.001). Table X shows the correlation between histological grade and the various histopronostic factors.

Table X: Histological grade and histopronostic factors

Grade histological			Location	Metastases	Perineural sheathing	Vascular emboli
	P	<0,001	0,16	0,12	0,14	0,46

111.10.2. Tumour stage and histopronostic parameters :

Tumour stage was positively correlated with tumour size, the presence of metastases and the presence of vascular emboli, as shown in Table XI.

Table XI: Tumour stage and histopronostic factors

Stadium tumor		Size	Location	Metastases	Perineural sheathing	Vascular emboli
	P	0,012	0,11	<0,001	0, 1^{19}	0,04

111.10.3. Tumour grade and stage :

We found no significant association between clinical stage and histological grade p=0.22.

111.10.4. Tumour size and metastases :

In our patients, tumour size was positively correlated with the presence of metastases. Tumour size greater than or equal to 30 mm was more associated with metastases (p=0.008).

111.10.5. Ki67 and tumour size :

Tumour size greater than or equal to 30 mm was significantly associated with a high Ki67, greater than 10% (p=0.037).

IV DISCUSSION

32

Digestive NETs are a heterogeneous group of tumours with histological and immunohistochemical features indicative of endocrine differentiation [1].

Fifty-five patients with a mean age of 43.4 years followed for digestive NETs were identified over a 12-year period from January 2005 to December 2016. They were 29 women and 26 men. The mean follow-up time was 51 months. At the end of the study and according to the history, physical examination and complementary examinations, the digestive NETs were distributed as follows: appendix 23 cases (41.8%), pancreas 8 cases (14.5%), graft intestine 7 cases (12.7%), stomach 6 cases (10.9%), duodenum 3 cases (5.4%), colon 1 case (1.8%), rectum 2 cases (3.6%), mesentery 2 cases (3.6%), hepatic location of unknown origin 3 cases (5.4%). The duration of clinical symptoms ranged from 3 days to 18 months, and varied according to location, with a clear predominance of abdominal pain (78.1%). Two patients presented with a flush syndrome. The extension work-up revealed hepatic metastases in 7 cases (12.7%): 3 hepatic metastases from an unknown primary and 4 metastatic primitives to the liver: 2 gall bladder NETs, 1 rectal NET and 1 pancreatic NET. Octreoscanner® showed distant neuroendocrine localisations in 3 cases. Anatomopathologically, all tumours were classified according to WHO 2010 grade and the UICC/AJCC TNM classification. Grade 1 clearly predominated: 54.5%. Two patients had mixed adeno-neuroendocrine carcinoma, which is a rare entity. Stage 1 was also the most frequent: 56.3%. Surgical treatment was indicated in 80% of cases, and was curative in 67.2% of cases. Tumour progression was noted in two cases, one of which was treated with somatostatin analogues and the other with adjuvant chemotherapy.

The mean survival in our patients was 51 months. Factors reducing survival in our patients were: grade 3, Ki67 greater than 10%, tumour size greater than 3 cm, poorly differentiated tumour, and presence of metastases. Advanced tumour grade (2 or 3) was significantly associated with the presence of metastases from all sites (p=0.007), and with no significant correlation with the presence of lymph node metastases (p=0.16). Tumour size, Ki67 value and mitotic index were positively correlated with the presence of metastases (p=0.008, p=0.009, p=0.004 respectively).

> **Workforce :**

1. We recruited the patients consecutively in a university hospital which drains a region with a large population. Consequently, our sample is representative of patients consulting in Tunisia.

2. This is the largest number of digestive NETs collected in a Tunisian series.

3. We have collected two cases of primary mesenteric NET, which is a very rare, if not exceptional, entity.

4. Our prognostic study revealed a positive correlation between tumour grade, tumour stage and the various histopronostic factors (size, site, presence of metastases), which underlines the importance of a good initial histological assessment for better therapeutic management.

> **Limits of the work :**

1. The small number of patients in some areas, such as the duodenum or colon.

2. The retrospective nature of work.

3. The large number of patients who were lost to follow-up hampered precise analysis of survival.

IV.1 Epidemiologic :

IV.1.1. Frequency :

NETs are rare tumours (1% of all tumours). In a Tunisian series published in 2016, 36 cases of digestive NETs among 1660 digestive tumours were identified, with a frequency of 2% [3].

The incidence of NETs is increasing, at 2 to 3 per 100,000 people per year, with a slight predominance of women.

In another epidemiological study carried out in Austria, the incidence of malignant digestive NETs was 0.8/100,000, but that of all NETs, benign and malignant, was 2.51/100,000 in men and 2.36/100,000 in women [4].

According to data from SEER (the Surveillance, Epidemiology and End Results Programme), and the NRC (the Norwegian Registry of Cancer), gastric and rectal tumours are becoming increasingly common, while the incidence of appendiceal NETs is declining [5, 6].

Other studies have reported an increase in this incidence between 1974 and 2004 from 2.1 to 9.3 new cases per 100,000 inhabitants per year [7].

In France, the incidence is rising and probably exceeds 1,000 new cases per year [8]. The incidence of appendiceal, caecal and pancreatic neuroendocrine tumours increased by a factor of 2 between 1975 and 2005. The incidence of rectal and gall bladder NETs increased by a factor of 4 during the same period, ranging from 0.9 to 1.3/100,000 patients/year [5, 6, 9]. In our series, digestive NETs represented 1.6% of all digestive tumours.

IV.1.2. Sex :

NETs are rarer before the age of 40 in both sexes, and their incidence then increases more rapidly in men than in women. Graft NETs are more common in men [10].

This was not consistent with the results of our series, which showed a slight female predominance (sex ratio: 0.85).

IV.1.3. Age :

The preferred age is between the fifth and sixth decade. The average age is 67 in men and 65 in women [8]. In another Italian study, the mean age was 51 [11]. In our series, the mean age of patients was 43.3 years.

IV.1.4 Epidemiology by location :

For well-differentiated NETs, the most common location is the grafted intestine, followed by the pancreas. In three French studies, jejunoileal tumours were the most common (21-43%), followed by duodenopancreatic NETs (21-36%), gastric NETs (611%), colonic and rectal NETs (13-27%), and appendicular NETs (5-8%). Other locations: gallbladder, liver, resophagus, peritoneum, are exceptional (<5%). In our series, appendicular location was the most frequent in approximately 41.8% of cases, followed by pancreatic location (14.5%) [8].

In another multicentre Austrian study, the locations were as follows: gastric (23.4%), duodenal (5.7%), pancreatic (11.9%), gallbladder (15.8%), appendicular (21.2%), colonic (7.2%) and rectal (14.8%) [12]. In a Tunisian series published in 2013, graft location was predominant in 30% of cases [13].

The gastric location was classified as 3eme in our series.

Table XII compares the epidemiological data from our study with three prospective French studies published in 2010 and 2011 [8].

Table XII: Epidemiological parameters compared with 3 French studies

	FFCD- ANGH- GERCOR	PRONET database	GTE basis	Our study
Year	2010	2011	2011	2016
Number of patients	668	778	2105	55
Sex ratio	1	1	0.9	0,85

Average age at diagnosis	56	61	50	**43**
Duodenum/Pancreas	32%	44%	49%	**20%**
Jejunum/ileon	43%	21%	27%	**12,7%**
Colon/Rectum	2%	13%	-	**5,4%**
Stomach	5%	11%	-	**10,9%**
Appendix	3%	8%	-	**41,8%**
Unknown	11%	3%	24%	**5,4%**

(FFCD: Federation française de cancerologie digestive, ANGH: Association des hepato-gastroenterologues des hopitaux generaux, GERCOR: Groupe cooperateur multidisciplinaire en oncologie, GTE: Groupe des tumeurs endocrines).

IV.2 Diagnosis :

IV.2.1. Clinical features :

A distinction is made between functional and non-functional NETs, depending on whether or not symptoms are associated with hormonal secretion by the tumour. Most digestive NETs are non-functional.

In a prospective series of 277 patients with GEP NETs published by Martin B et al, abdominal pain was the main symptom in 29.5% of cases, followed by diarrhoea (8.7%) and weight loss in 7.5% of cases [12]. In our series, abdominal pain was also the most frequent symptom (78.1%), with alteration in general condition observed in 11.5% of cases.

Functional NETs are revealed by symptoms which depend on the type of hormone secreted, as shown in table XIII [14] :

Table XIII: Clinical presentation of functional NETs according to the hormone secreted [14].

Tumour	Symptoms
Insulinoma	Confusion, sweating, dizziness, asthenia, loss of consciousness, improvement after a meal.
Gastrinoma	Severe peptic ulceration and diarrhoea, or isolated diarrhoea
Glucagonoma	Migratory necrolytic erythema, weight loss, diabetes, stomatitis, diarrhoea
VIPome	Verner-Morrison syndrome with profuse diarrhoea and hypokalemia
Somatostatinoma	Cholelithiasis, weight loss, diarrhoea and steatorrhea, diabetes
Non-syndromic pancreatic NETs	Symptoms associated with pancreatic mass effect or hepatic metastases

In our series, only one NET was highly likely to be functional (gastrinoma). Functionality was suspected in view of the suggestive appearance on octreoscan and the presence of multiple resophageal, gastric and duodenal ulcerations on upper gastrointestinal endoscopy.

IV.2.1.1. Carcinoid syndrome :

It is seen in 20% of well-differentiated ileal and juvenile NETs, and more frequently in cases of associated hepatic metastases.

It typically associates a flush (a paroxysmal vasomotor erythema of the face, neck and anterior chest), without associated sweating in 70% of cases [15], diarrhoea in 50% of cases, and intermittent abdominal pain in 40% of cases. Symptoms may appear spontaneously, but are often triggered by an emotion, physical exercise, certain foods or the intake of alcohol in 70% of cases [16].

Two patients in our series presented with flush syndrome, 1 with appendicular NET[er] and 2 with hepatic metastases of unknown origin .[eme]

IV.2.1.2. Carcinogenic heart disease :

It is linked to fibrous thickening of the endocardium of the right heart [17]. It is manifested by valvular damage in the form of tricuspid insufficiency, and is responsible for the death of patients in 1/3 of cases.

Cardiac ultrasound was performed in only 5 patients and revealed signs of tricuspid insufficiency in one.

IV.2.2. Clinical presentation by site :

IV. 2.2.1. NETs (Esophageal :

The presence of an associated endobrachyoesophagus (EBO) is common [18]. Dysphagia or gatsro-oesophageal reflux symptoms are usually revelatory. More rarely, a complication such as digestive haemorrhage may occur.

In our series, no cases of resophageal NET were reported.

IV.2.2.2. Gastric NETs :

The clinical presentation is highly variable, and may include abdominal pain, vomiting, upper GI haemorrhage or carcinoid syndrome [19]. In most cases, it is discovered incidentally during the investigation of anaemia. In our series, the main presenting sign was abdominal pain in 80% of cases.

IV. 2.2.3. Grafted NETs :

They may present with abdominal pain, or be complicated by intestinal obstruction requiring urgent surgery. In the case of secreting tumours, they may manifest as a carcinoid syndrome [20, 21]. In our series, the tumour was revealed by an occlusive syndrome in 2 cases.

IV.2.2.4. Pancreatic NETs :

In about half the cases, the symptoms are dominated by the mass effect of the tumour: abdominal pain, icterus, etc. Symptoms may also be associated with hormonal hypersecretion: recurrent hypoglycaemia, high blood sugar levels, multiple gastric or duodenal ulcers associated with gastrinoma, etc. [22, 23].

In our series, the tumour was revealed by an epigastric mass in 2 cases and abdominal pain with an alteration in general condition in 6 cases (75%).

IV.2.2.5. Colonic NETs :

Caecal location is the most common [24]. The most common symptoms are transit disorders (especially diarrhoea), abdominal pain and, rarely, acute intestinal obstruction. Carcinoid syndrome is rare in this location [25]. In our series, the only case of a right colonic tumour presented with a sub-occlusive syndrome and chronic anaemia. Its location was caecal, consistent with the literature.

IV.2.2.6. Rectal NETs :

In around 50% of cases, the tumour is discovered by chance during a colonoscopy. Bowel movements and rectal syndrome may reveal these tumours. Carcinoid syndrome is exceptional. In an American study of 85 patients, the tumour was asymptomatic in 39% of cases, 22% of patients had rectal discharge and 8% had rectal syndrome [26].

In our series, one rectal NET was revealed by anal pain and another by rectal discharge and anaemia.

IV.3. Biology :

Biological parameters are used for diagnostic and prognostic purposes. Bioactive peptides are secreted by functional and non-functional tumours:

IV.3.1. Chromogranin A :

Elevated levels of circulating chromogranin A are observed in 60-80% of cases of digestive NETs in both functional and non-functional tumours [27], and its level may correlate with tumour size. In our series, chromogranin "A" was measured in 5 patients and was elevated in 4 of them.

IV.3.2. Urinary 5-hydroxyindole acetic acid (5-HIAA) :

It is a serotonin metabolite excreted in the urine. It has a sensitivity of 50-70% for diagnosing intestinal NETs and a specificity of 90-100%, especially in cases of hepatic metastases or carcinoid syndrome. It has prognostic value, as high levels of urinary 5-HIAA are associated with a more guarded prognosis; it also serves as a means of post-therapeutic monitoring. Urinary 5-HIAA was measured in a single patient with hepatic metastases from an unrecognised primary and was elevated to 38 times normal.

IV.3.3. Specific hormones :

They are responsible for the clinical symptoms of functional tumours [28]. Table XIV illustrates the specific hormonal markers and biological parameters of the different functional NETs [21] :

Table XIV: Hormonal syndromes and specific markers of functional NETs [21].

Hormonal syndromes	Hormone/peptide	Biological manifestations
Carcinoid syndrome	Serotonin, Histamine, Dopamine, Prostaglandins, Tachykinins	Elevation of urinary 5 HIAA
Insulinoma	Insulin	Hypoglycaemia associated with high blood concentrations of insulin, pro-insulin and C-peptide
Zollinger-Ellison syndrome	Gastrin	Fasting hypergastrinemia, elevated basal acid flow, secretin test
VIPome (Verner-Morrison syndrome)	VIP	Elevation of plasma VIP, Hypokalemia, Hypochlorhydria, Metabolic acidosis
Glucagonoma	Glucagon	Elevation of plasma glucagon, Hyperglycemia, Anemia

IV.4 Endoscopy :

The various endoscopic examinations (upper digestive endoscopy, colonoscopy) are used to diagnose gastric and colorectal NETs, and rarely NETs of the last ileal appendages.

IV.4.1. EOGD :

It is used to diagnose NETs from the resophagus to the Treitz angle (Tsophagus, stomach, duodenum). Image 14 shows a bulbar NET.

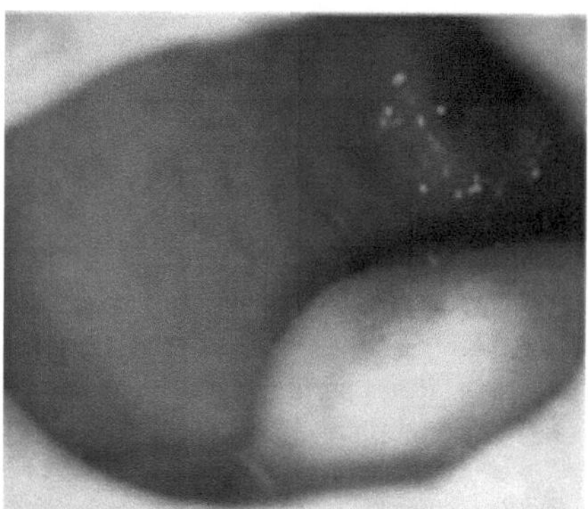
Image 14: Endoscopic bulbar NET

In the resophagus, NETs are most frequently found in the lower third. Duodenal localisation is rare; in this case, tumours are usually seen in the bulb, the 2eme duodenum or the papilla. In a Chinese study highlighting the value of EOGD in the diagnosis of NETs of the upper GI tract, 13 cases of NETs were found incidentally: 1 case of resophageal, 9 gastric and 3 duodenal NETs, with a polypoid or submucosal appearance [29]. The endoscopic findings of our series are consistent with the literature, as we found one case of ampullary localisation confirmed by echoendoscopy, and one case of bulbar NET in the form of polypoid formations. Gastric NETs were polypoid in 4 out of 5 cases.

IV.4.2. Colonoscopy :

NETs of the hindgut are often rectal in origin. However, total colonoscopy is indicated when associated with colonic adenocarcinoma, which can account for up to 20% of cases. Rectosigmoidoscopy usually reveals these tumours as single polypoid sessile formations, sometimes ulcerated [30]. Image 15 shows a rectal NET on endoscopy.

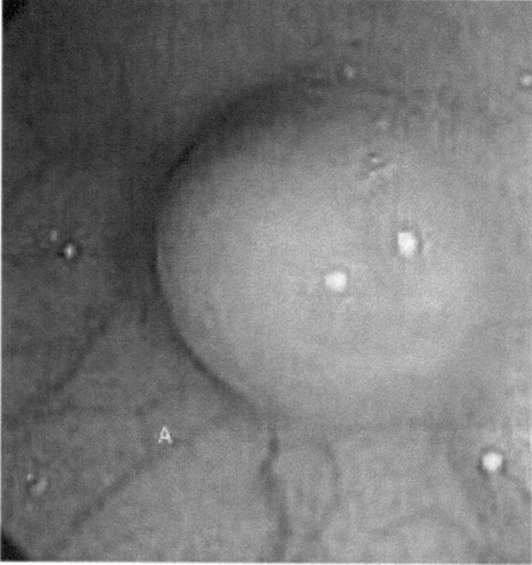

Image 15: Endoscopic appearance of a rectal NET < 1 cm

In our series, ileocolonoscopy identified tumours in 4 cases: an ulcerating tumour process in the lower caecal fundus, a submucosal formation in the middle rectum, a sessile polyp in the middle rectum, and a polypoid formation 35 mm in diameter in the last loop of the ileum.

IV.4.3. Endoscopic videocapsule :

It has been shown to be effective in diagnosing grafted NETs [31, 32]. Its sensitivity ranges from 42 to 76%. The risk of incarceration limits its indications, despite its efficacy in detecting grafted NETs.

In our work, none of the patients underwent videocapsule exploration.

IV.4.4 Echoendoscopy :

Echoendoscopy is an operative-dependent examination which remains useful in small duodeno-pancreatic NETs (especially insulinomas and gastrinomas) with a sensitivity of 79 to 94%; sensitivity is better in the head than in the tail of the pancreas [42]. It can also be used to assess locoregional invasion of the tumour.

Two patients with an ampullary NET and a NET of the head of the pancreas were explored by echoendoscopy in our series.

IV.5 Imaging :

The morphological work-up has a triple purpose: diagnostic, as part of the pre-therapeutic work-up and post-therapeutic monitoring. This work-up is guided by the clino-biological characteristics of the primary tumour.

Combining conventional imaging with functional imaging (octreoscan and PET scan) improves the sensitivity of these tests.

IV.5.1. Abdominal ultrasound :

It remains an essential test, given its safety and availability. Its main benefit is the detection of hepatic metastases, and it can be used to guide biopsies of metastases when the primary is unknown. Tumours can take on different appearances on ultrasound: hypo- or hyper-echogenic, or heterogenic.

Its sensitivity is low for the detection of primary NETs but increases to 38% for hepatic metastases [33].

In our series, ultrasound was useful in the diagnosis of hepatic metastases where it objectified a multinodular liver in 6 cases and allowed biopsy of the hepatic metastases for diagnostic confirmation. A primary NET was visualised in 13 cases: 2 pancreatic NETs, one jejunal NET, 2 mesenteric NETs, 1 NET in the form of a nodule in the back cavity of the epiplons, 6 cases of appendicular NETs and one colonic NET.

IV.5.2. Computed tomography :

CT is an essential test for diagnosing gastroenteropancreatic NETs and their metastases, especially in the liver. Its sensitivity in detecting primary tumours varies from 60 to 90% depending on the site [34].

The typical appearance is a hypodense tumour that becomes hyperdense after injection of contrast, in keeping with the hypervascular nature of these tumours. Less typical features may include nodular calcifications, heterogeneous contrast and fibrosis with retraction of the mesentery [35, 36].

In our study, a CT scan was performed in approximately half of the cases. It identified the primary tumour in 21 cases: 6 cases of NET of the graft, 8 pancreatic NETs, 2 mesenteric NETs, two duodenal tumours (ampulla of Vater), one colonic NET, one rectal NET and one gastric NET. Hepatic metastases were observed in 7 cases. A typical appearance was noted in 12.7% of our patients.

IV.5.3 Magnetic resonance imaging :

The diagnostic performance of magnetic resonance imaging (MRI) is identical to or even better than that of CT in certain locations, especially in the gallbladder and pancreas [37-39]. Its sensitivity reaches 94% in pancreatic locations, and is lower in extra-pancreatic NETs [38,

40].

MRI is superior to CT in detecting liver and bone metastases.

Typically, these tumours have a T1 hypersignal and a T2 hypersignal [41]. They are

generally detected on the sequence with T1 fat saturation, hypo signal compared with the surrounding parenchyma.

In our series, additional MRI was used to support the diagnosis in 3 cases: 2 cases of pancreatic NETs and 1 case of grafted NET with hepatic metastases.

IV.5.4. Octreoscanner® :

The majority of well-differentiated NETs express somatostatin receptors on their surface, which can be detected by the binding of a radioactive analogue with a longer half-life than somatostatin: lanreotide and octreotide. In fact, the majority of digestive and pancreatic neuroendocrine tumours and their metastases, with the exception of insulinoma, express these receptors. Other tumours that may express RSS include pituitary adenomas, paragangliomas, pheochromocytomas, small cell lung carcinomas, medullary thyroid cancer, breast carcinomas and malignant lymphomas.

Octreoscanner® is currently recommended for the extension assessment of any well-differentiated NET. Its sensitivity varies from 57 to 93% depending on the type of tumour and its location [43, 44], and is low for tumours smaller than 1 cm. Functional NETs are better detected than non-functional tumours (detection rate 82% versus 73%). It is much less sensitive for non-differentiated NETs [45, 46]. This was demonstrated by Malcolm H et al [47]. In an American study published in the Annals of Surgical Oncology, the sensitivity of octreoscanner® was around 80% for grade 1 and 2 NETs with no significant difference compared with FDG PET, which was significantly more sensitive than octreoscanner for grade 3 NETs [47].

In our series, an octreoscanner® was performed in 17 cases and found to be remotely located in 4 cases.

IV.5.5. PET Scan :

Binderup et al demonstrated an overall sensitivity of PET scan of around 60% in a cohort of 96 patients with gastro-entero-pancreatic NETs [48]. It outperforms octreoscan in the diagnosis of well-differentiated NETs with high Ki67 (>10%). FDG-TEP-Scan is therefore indicated if RSS scintigraphy is negative or if Ki67 is greater than 10%, and as a first-line treatment for neuroendocrine carcinoma with a low degree of differentiation [28].

Its disadvantage is its limited availability, even in developed countries [49].

In our series, no patient was explored by this examination.

IV.6 Anatomopathology :

IV.6.1. Type of sampling :

IV.6.1.1. Endoscopic or radiologically guided biopsies :

Their deep mucosal and submucosal location, as well as their small size, make the diagnosis of NETs on biopsy material rather difficult. In fact, this material may not contain enough cells for Ki67 or mitotic index to be established, leading to diagnostic errors.

In a Tunisian series published in 2013, the positive diagnosis was made by biopsy in 15.6% [13]. In a Moroccan series published in 2011, involving 14 patients with digestive NETs, ultrasound-guided biopsy was used in 42.8% of cases [50].

In our series, tumour sampling by endoscopic biopsy was performed in 11 cases. It was positive in all cases.

Ultrasound-guided biopsy was performed in 4 cases (7.2%).

IV.6.1.2. Anatomopathological study on the operating room :

In our study, 44 tumour samples were obtained from surgical resection specimens, either in an emergency setting (appendectomy for appendicular syndrome, for example) or scheduled surgery with a full pre-therapeutic work-up prior to surgery.

IV.6.2. Macroscopy :

Macroscopic assessment of the tumour reveals its location, size, whether it is single or multiple, its appearance (solid/cystic), the presence of necrosis and its degree of invasion or extension.

The macroscopic appearance depends on the site and grade of the tumour.

IV.6.2.1. Pancreatic NETs :

In the pancreas, NETs are distributed in equal proportions between the head, body and tail. Glucagonomas, vipomas and insulinomas tend to be located in the body or tail of the pancreas, gastrinomas and non-functional tumours more often in the head, and somatostatinomas in the periampullary zone.

Pancreatic NETs are usually unique, except when they develop as part of a genetic disease (NEM1) [51].

In our patients, the tumour was unique in all cases. A cephalic pancreatic location was noted in 4 cases and a left pancreatic location in 4 cases (50%).

IV.6.2.2. Gastric NETs :

There are 4 types: NETs with ECL1, 2 and 3 cells and non-ECL tumours. The macroscopic appearance varies according to the type of tumour. ECL1 and 2 are generally small, polypoid and multiple. ECL3 and non-ECL NETs are single, larger and invasive [51].

In our series, there were 4 type 1 gastric NETs and a single type 2 NET. Multiple polypoid formations were seen in 2 patients.

IV.6.2.3. Duodenal NETs :

They often have a small, ampullary seat. The WHO classifies duodenal and ampullary NETs in the same category, but numerous recent studies have shown that these 2 entities differ histologically [52]: ampullary NETs are more aggressive and express more somatostatin. Neurofibromatosis may be associated with 25% of cases of ampullary NETs, but is very rare in duodenal NETs [53]. Macroscopically, they occur more frequently in the first portion of the duodenum (D1) and their frequency decreases with distance from D1 [54]. In our series, 3 patients had a duodenal location: bulbar in 1 case and ampullary in two cases.

IV. 6.2.4. Gallic NETs:

They are generally small, and multiple in 30% of cases. They are usually located in the terminal ileum [9, 55].

In our series, only one patient (1.8%) had a double location and only one patient (1.8%) had involvement of the terminal ileum.

IV.6.2.5. Appendicular NETs :

Always small in size, they are often associated with lesions of acute appendicitis or chronic obliterative appendicitis. They are most frequently located at the tip [56]. In our series, NET was located at the tip in 20 cases (87%), which is consistent with the literature.

IV.6.2.6. Colonic NETs :

They may be polypoid, covered by normal mucosa, infiltrative or even circumferential and obstructive. Larger tumours may be ulcerated [24].

In our series, the colonic tumour was on the right, with an ulcerobourgeous appearance.

IV.6.2.7. Rectal NETs :

They present as small multiple polypoid lesions, either sessile or rounded [57]. Our results for the rectal location are similar to those reported in the literature concerning the macroscopic appearance: a sessile polyp in 1 case, and a non-ulcerated submucosal formation in the second case.

IV.6.3. Microscopy :

NET-GEPs have a lobular or trabecular architecture, with a stroma that varies in abundance but is always hypervascularised. The endocrine tumour cells have a very stereotyped appearance: they are monomorphic and medium-sized, with a nucleus with fine chromatin in a central position and abundant cytoplasm with a clear boundary.

IV. 6.3.1. Degree of differentiation :

- **Differentiated NETs :**

Well differentiated NETs have histological and immunohistochemical characteristics similar to normal neuroendocrine cells. The cells are monomorphic, polygonal, small to medium-sized, with abundant eosinophilic cytoplasm and sharp borders. Their nuclei are regular, rounded or ovoid, with clumped chromatin. The nucleolus is usually invisible. Cytonuclear atypia are not very marked.

Tumour proliferation can have a variable architecture: insular, trabecular or acinar [58].

The mitotic index is an essential element in the classification of these tumours, and is studied on at least 50 fields at high magnification (2 mm^2 according to the WHO) and expressed for ten fields. The mitotic index is less than 2 in G1 NETs and between 2 and 20 in G2 NETs.

In our series, well-differentiated NETs predominated (92.7%).

- **Not very differentiated NETs:**

The cellular architecture is generally in the form of clusters or sheets, and is sometimes trabecular or rosette-shaped [59]. Depending on the size of the tumour cells, we distinguish 2 types: large-cell and small-cell tumours. Nuclear atypia is common, and the mitotic index is generally high. Vascular emboli and sheathing are more common than in well-differentiated NETs.

In our series, 2 cases of NETs of little difference were noted: a colonic NET and a grafted NET, both tumours were large-cell.

IV.6.3.2. Immunohistochemical study :

– Differentiation markers :

Two markers are needed to confirm the neuroendocrine nature of a tumour. Chromogranin A and synaptophysin are generally used as they are the most specific. If one of the markers is negative, CD56 is used.

– There are 4 types of marker:

-> Markers associated with secretory granules: chromogranins, a highly specific marker for neuroendocrine tumour cells. The most commonly used is chromogranin A. A Japanese study published by Masayuki et al demonstrated the value of chromogranin A in the diagnosis of pancreatic NETs; this marker was significantly higher in patients with pancreatic NETs than in those with chronic pancreatitis or adenocarcinoma [60]. The results of our series confirm this notion of specificity, given that 80% of our patients were positive for chromogranin A and 87.5% of pancreatic NETs were positive for this marker.

^ Markers associated with secretory vesicles: especially synaptophysin, which is expressed more in grade 2 and 3 NETs than in G1 NETs according to two studies published by Al-Khafaji et al and Rindi et al [61, 62]. In our series, this marker was positive in 72.7% of cases. Contrary to the literature, synaptophysin was expressed as frequently in G1 NETs as in G2 and 3 NETs (50%).

^ Cytosolic markers: NSE (Neuron Specific Enolase), not very specific for neuroendocrine cells.

-> Membrane markers: the best known is N-CAM (neural-cell adhesion molecule).

In our series, NSE and N-CAM were not used in any cases. Positive labelling for CD56 and CK7 was observed in 10 and 8 cases respectively. These two markers were used when labelling was negative for chromogranin A (n=11) or synaptophysin (n=16).

- Ki67 proliferation index:

This is an important prognostic factor, particularly since 2006 when ENETS proposed the determination of a histological grade for endocrine carcinomas based on the combination of the mitotic index and the Ki-67 proliferation index [63, 64]. This is assessed by immunohistochemistry using the MIB1 antibody (which recognises the Ki-67 protein expressed by tumour cells), followed by a count of labelled cells per 2000 cells in the areas of highest cell density. Grade 1 neuroendocrine tumours have a proliferation index of less than 3%, and grade 3 NETs have a Ki-67 of more than 20%.

In our series, the average Ki-67 was 5% and exceeded 20% in 6 cases.

IV.6.3.3. Mitotic index :

The mitotic index is a key prognostic factor in the WHO 2010 classification. Its main limitation is its lack of reproducibility. It depends on the thickness of the sections, the intensity of the staining and the antibody used. Its determination does not require any particular technique, but can only be applied to a sample of sufficient size. The literature is patchy on the complementarity of Ki67 and the mitotic index (MI) in determining tumour grade. A study published by Strosberg et al showed a good correlation between the 2 indices [65], whereas MS Khan et al emphasised the superiority of Ki67 as a prognostic factor in metastatic NETs [66].

In our series, the mean MI was 3 mitoses per CFG. We found a good correlation between Ki67 and MI, which is consistent with the results of Strosberg et al.

IV.6.3.4 Histological grade and classifications :

- WHO 2000/2010:

Digestive NETs were included in the World Health Organisation (WHO) classification for the first time in 2000. This classification was completed in 2004 with that of the pancreas.

In 2010, the WHO updated this classification and introduced several changes. The philosophy of the new classification is based around three main axes [67, 68]:

^ A clear distinction between histological classification and staging.

-> To underline the existence of a risk of malignancy inherent in any well-differentiated neuroendocrine tumour.

^ The clinical importance of histological grading

Table XV shows the correspondence between the WHO 2000 and 2010 classifications of digestive NETs [69].

Table XV: Correspondence between the WHO 2000 classification and the WHO 2010 classification
of digestive endocrine tumours.

WHO 2010	WHO 2000
G1 neuroendocrine tumour G2 neuroendocrine tumour Small cell neuroendocrine carcinoma	• Endocrine tumour well differentiated from benign behaviour. • Well differentiated endocrine tumour of uncertain behaviour with mitotic index < 2 and Ki67 < or equal to 2%. • Well differentiated endocrine carcinoma with mitotic index < 2

Large cell neuroendocrine carcinoma Mixed adeno-neuroendocrine carcinoma	and Ki67 index < or equal to 2%. • Well differentiated endocrine tumour of uncertain behaviour with a mitotic index of between 2 and 20 and/or a Ki67 index of between 3 and 20%. • Well differentiated endocrine carcinoma with a mitotic index of between 2 and 20 and/or a Ki67 index of between 3 and 20%. • Poorly differentiated small cell carcinoma • No corresponding category • Mixed tumour

It should be noted that a new 2017 WHO classification for the pancreas has distinguished two G3 subgroups: G3 well/moderately differentiated and G3 poorly differentiated. This classification already supersedes the WHO 2010 classification for all other digestive tract sites [70]. The following table illustrates the 2017 WHO classification and the differences compared with the previous classification (Table XVI).

Table XVI: 2017 WHO classification of pancreatic NETs

	WHO 2010	WHO 2017
G1	Well/moderately differentiated neuroendocrine tumour Ki67 0-2	Well/moderately differentiated neuroendocrine tumour Ki67 0-2.99
G2	Well/moderately differentiated neuroendocrine tumour Ki67 2-20	Well/moderately differentiated neuroendocrine tumour Ki67 3-20
G3	Poorly differentiated neuroendocrine carcinoma	- **Well/moderately differentiated neuroendocrine tumour G3** - Poorly differentiated neuroendocrine carcinoma G3
Mixed tumour	MANEC: Mixed adenoneuroendocrine carcinoma	MiNEN: Mixed endocrine and non-endocrine neoplasia

Juha Jernman et al, in a study published in 2012, demonstrated the contribution of the 2010 WHO classification compared with that of 2000 in assessing the malignant potential of metastatic rectal NETs: 5 rectal NETs were classified as low-grade malignant according to the 2000 WHO classification and G2 according to that of 2010; only grade 2 and 3 NETs were metastatic (p<0.001) [71]. In our series, of the 10 metastatic NETs, 2 were classified as grade 1 according to the 2010 WHO classification. A correlation study between WHO grade and the presence of metastases showed a non-significant correlation (p = 0.12).

- TNM classification and clinical stage :

This classification was devised under the aegis of TENETS and was first published in 2006, and completed in 2007 for tumours of the mid- and hindgut. Subsequently, a TNM classification appeared in 2009 [72], officially proposed by the UICC (International Union Against Cancer), which depends on the site of the tumour.

The WHO currently recommends the classification proposed by the UICC/AJCC.

In 2012, the UK and Ireland Neuroendocrine Tumor Society (UKI NETS) recommended the 7th edition AJCC or tumour site specific ENETS classification for stomach, pancreas and appendix [14]. In our series, cases were classified according to TNM 7me edition. This classification was updated in 2017 [70] (Appendix 4).

Figure 17 shows the different classifications and when they were created.

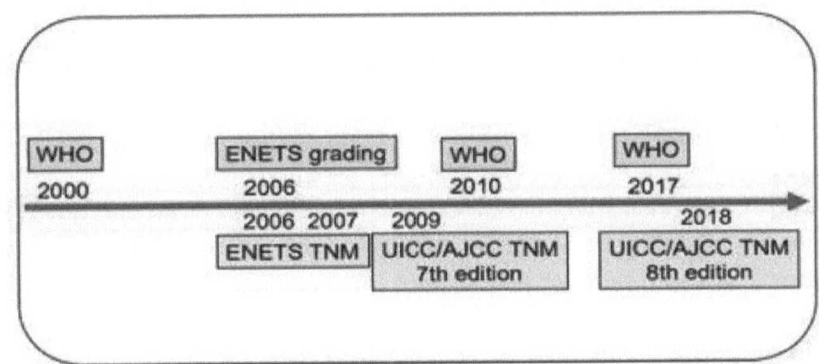

Figure 17: Recent history and future of digestive NET classifications

Gastric NETs are most often localised at the time of diagnosis [4].

Pancreatic NETs are most often metastatic at diagnosis, with stage 4 observed in more than 40% of cases in some series [73]. In a recent Chinese study published by Min Yang et al, 145 patients with pancreatic NETs were enrolled, with the following stages: stage I: 57.9%, stage II: 26.2%, stage III: 8.2%, stage IV: 7.7% [74]. In our series, stage IV was noted in only one case (12.5%).

Stage IV is observed in 50 to 77% of cases of graft NETs, and metastases are frequent. Appendiceal NETs are most often stage I or II at diagnosis. In a study published by Paula B et al, involving 93 patients, intestinal NETs (including appendicular NETs) were divided into: stage I: 8.6%, stage II: 8.6%, stage III: 39.8% and stage IV: 43% [75]. In our series, 2 grafted NETs were stage IV (28.5%).

Colonic NETs are stage IV at diagnosis in around 40% of cases. Rectal NETs are frequently stage I at diagnosis. In a Core study of 514 colonic (n=14) and rectal (n=500) NETs, the tumours were divided into: stage I: 93.8%, stage II: 0.9%, stage III: 4.8% and stage IV: 0.5% [76].

In our series, colonic NET was classified as stage III and rectal NET as stages II and IV, which is inconsistent with the literature. Table XVII shows the distribution of TNM stages according to site in different studies.

Table XVII: Distribution of TNM stages by site

Location	Serie	Number of cases	Stage I	Stadium II	Stage III	Stage IV
Grele + Appendix	Paula B et al [75]	93	8.6%	8.6%	39.8%	43%
	Our series	**29**	**75,8%**	**13,7%**	**3,4%**	**7,1%**
Colon + Rectum	Korean Society of Coloproctology [76]	514	93.8%	0.9%	4.8%	0.5%
	3	**0%**	**33%**	**33%**	**33%**
	Our series					
Pancreas	Min Yang et al [74]	145	57.9%	26.2%	8.2%	7.7%
	Our series	**8**	**37,5%**	**50%**	**0%**	**12,5%**

IV.7. Therapeutic management :

The therapeutic approach depends mainly on the histological nature of the tumour and the type of hormone secretion.

Differentiated NETs are subject to either surveillance, surgery or systemic chemotherapy.

Neuroendocrine carcinomas are generally treated with chemotherapy and have a favourable prognosis.

IV.7.1. Medical treatment :

IV.7.1.1 Symptomatic treatment :

Treatment of the symptoms associated with tumour secretion is essential. It depends on the type of tumour secretion.

PPIs are indicated in cases of Zollinger-Ellison syndrome. The initial dose is 60mg/d. Three patients in our series were started on PPIs and their symptoms improved.

Diazoxide: Diazoxide is indicated in insulinoma with an efficacy of around 50% [77]. Thirty to fifty percent of patients with insulinoma may improve on diazoxide, but this must be strictly monitored, as the treatment may worsen the condition. None of our patients were put on this treatment.

Somatostatin analogues: indicated in carcinoid syndrome, symptomatic glucagonoma and VIPoma.

In fact, somatostatin is a natural hormone present in the endocrine cells of the gastrointestinal tract and in the D cells of the pancreatic islets.

It reduces the serum concentration of numerous intestinal peptides (insulin, glucagon, gastrin, etc.) and inhibits the postprandial physiological response to these peptides. Its half-life is only a few minutes, which limits its therapeutic use. Analogues with a high affinity for the sst2 and sst5 receptors have been developed (octreotide: Sandostatin®, Lanreotide: Somatuline®). Delayed-acting forms of these analogues have the advantage of requiring only one monthly or fortnightly injection, which improves compliance, comfort and quality of life for patients undergoing treatment. A recent prospective study (PROMID) showed the efficacy of Sandostatin LAR in metastatic midgut NET with a progression-free survival (PFS) of 1.3 months compared with 6 months in the placebo group [78]. In our series, 6 patients with hepatic and lymph node metastases were treated with somatostatin analogues. The PFS was 8.16 months (compared with 14 months in the literature).

IV.7.1.2 Interferon :

This molecule has a dual effect: anti-secretory and anti-tumour. It is used in the treatment of functional and non-functional NETs, with or without somatostatin analogues which can be combined to increase the anti-tumour effect [79]. An increase in the 5-year survival rate with interferon and octreotide compared with interferon alone was noted in a single study (57% versus 37%) [80]. The recommended dose is 3 to 5 MIU, 3 to 5 days a week, subcutaneously. Improvement in symptoms can be seen in 40 to 60% of cases, with tumour reduction in 10 to 15% of patients.

Interferon has been shown to be more effective in tumours with a low mitotic index [81]. It is used as a 2®^{me} line therapy when other medical treatments have failed. In our series, no patient received interferon.

IV.7.1.3. Targeted therapies :

New therapeutic options have recently been proposed, in particular Sunitinib and Everolimus.

- **Sunitinib**

Sunitinib is a tyrosine kinase receptor inhibitor with anti-tumour and anti-angiogenic activity. It is indicated in locally advanced or metastatic neuroendocrine tumours. A study published by Raymond et al assessed the efficacy of sunitinib in patients with well-differentiated pancreatic NETs who had progressed according to RECIST criteria over the previous 12 months. The authors compared two groups of patients: one on sunitinib and the other on placebo. Both groups were treated concomitantly with somatostatin analogues. Progression-free survival (PFS) was significantly better in the sunitinib arm (11.1 months versus 5.5 months) [82]. In our series, no patient received this treatment.

- **Everolimus :**

It is an inhibitor of mTOR (mammalian Target Of Rapamycin), which is involved in cell proliferation and angiogenesis. A multicentre randomised study (RADIANT II) compared Everolimus 10 mg/d to placebo combined with octreotide LP 30 mg every 4 weeks. Progression-free survival was better in the Everolimus arm with a significant difference (16.4 versus 11.3 months) [83]. None of the patients in our series received Everolimus.

- **Bevacizumab :**

Bevacizumab is an IgG1 monoclonal antibody that binds to VEGF (vascular endothelial growth factor) and has an anti-angiogenic effect. A French phase 2 study (BETTER) evaluated the place of a combination of chemotherapy and Bevacizumab in the treatment of advanced and progressive differentiated digestive neuroendocrine tumours. Tumour control was obtained in 87% of cases for tumours of the digestive tract and 100% for duodeno-pancreatic NETs [84]. None of the patients in our series received this treatment.

IV.7.1.4. Systemic chemotherapy :

Chemotherapy is the reference treatment if the main objective is tumour reduction.

It is indicated in non-resectable G3 NETs, progressive non-resectable pancreatic NETs and metastatic gastro-duodeno-pancreatic NETs. For pancreatic NETs, treatment is based on regimens including Streptozotocin + Doxorubicin or Streptozotocin + 5 FU with an objective response rate of 40 to 70% and an overall median survival of more than 2 years [85]. In a randomised phase 3 study, Dahan et al compared the efficacy of Streptozotocin-5FU versus Interferon in 64 patients with non-pancreatic digestive NETs, and the two groups were comparable in terms of overall survival (OS) and progression-free survival (PFS) [86]. In our series, chemotherapy was indicated in 6 cases. Progression-free survival in our patients was 10.6 months.

Table XVIII and diagrams 1 and 2 illustrate the recommended uses of the various anti-tumour drugs in advanced NET in P[re] [87].

Table XVIII: Indications for somatostatin analogues, targeted therapies and chemotherapy (CT) in locally advanced or metastatic pancreatic NETs

Medication	Grade	Location of the primitive	SSTR status	Special considerations and indications
Octreotide	G1	Midgut	+	Low tumour load
Lanreotide	**G1/G2**	Midgut, **pancreas**	+	High tumour load (>25%) and low tumour load in the liver
STZ/5-FU	G1/G2	Pancreas		Rapid progression (<6 months) or high or symptomatic tumour burden
TEM/CAP	G2	Pancreas		Rapid progression or high or symptomatic tumour burden; when STZ is contraindicated or not available
Everolimus	G1/G2	Pancreas Midgut		Atypical carcinoid and/or negative SSTR;
				insulinoma or contraindication to CT if SSTR is negative
Sunitinib	G1/G2	Pancreas		Contraindication to CT
Cisplatin/Etoposide	G3	All locations		All CNEs are slightly

		combined		different

(STZ: Streptozotocin, 5-FU: 5 Fluo uracil, TEM/CAP: Temozolomide-Capecitabine, CT: Chemotherapy, SSTR: Somatostatin Receptor, CNE: Neuroendocrine Carcinoma)

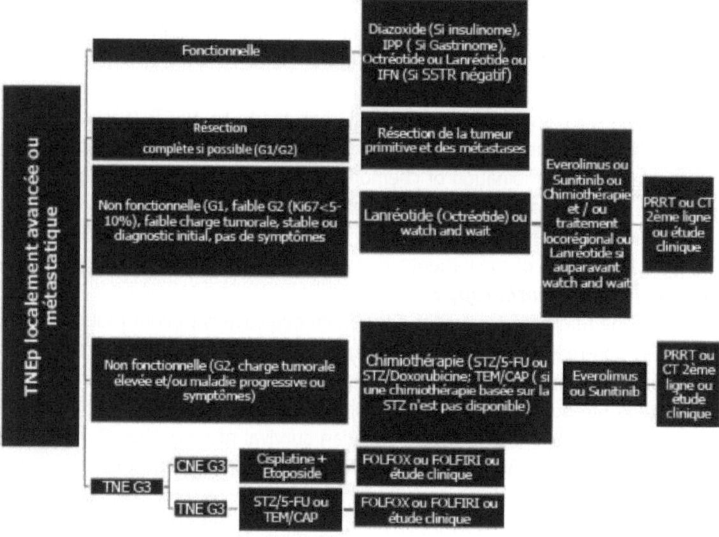

Schema 1: Management of locally advanced or metastatic pancreatic NETs (Regardless of secondary location) (: Tumor progression) [87]

(IFN: Interferon, SSTR: Somatostatin Receptor, STZ: Streptozotocin, 5-FU: 5 Fluo uracil, TEM/CAP: Temozolomide-Capecitabine, PRRT: Peptide Receptor Radionuclide Therapy)

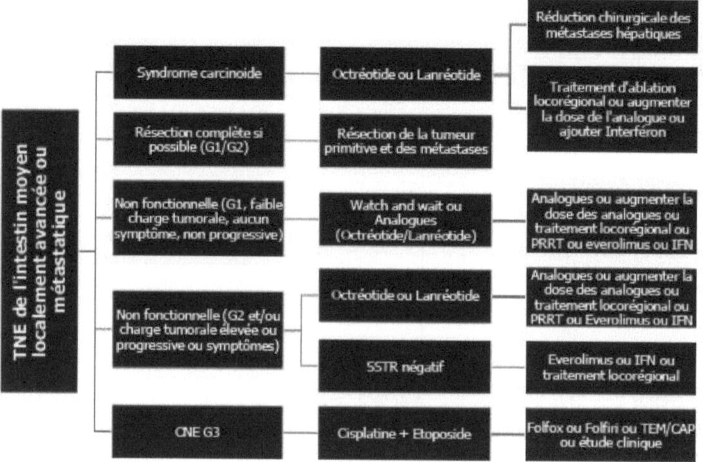

Schema 2: Management of locally advanced or metastatic NETs of the grafted bowel (midgut) (regardless of secondary location) (: carcinoid syndrome

48

refractory ;   : Tumour progression)
(SSTR: Somatostatin Receptor, IFN: Interferon, PRRT: Peptide Receptor Radionuclide Therapy, TEM/CAP: Temozolomide-Capecitabine)

IV.7.2. Targeted nuclear therapies :

NETs in inoperable patients who are locally advanced or remain symptomatic and are progressing on somatostatin analogues or chemotherapy are a good indication for targeted nuclear therapy. No randomised controlled trials have been performed to evaluate these therapies in digestive NETs. None of our patients has undergone targeted nuclear therapy.

IV.7.3. Radiological treatment

IV.7.3.1. Hepatic arterial chemo embolisation :

It is indicated for the treatment of symptomatic, non-resectable G1 and G2 hepatic metastases [88, 89]. Several studies have reported the benefit of this therapeutic modality in terms of survival and tumour control. Tumour response is obtained in approximately 50% of cases [90, 91].

Mortality at 30 days post-embolisation ranges from 1.9% to 9.3% [14], hence the importance of careful patient selection for the best results. The mortality rate is higher in patients with more than 75% hepatic parenchymal involvement, portal thrombosis and carcinoid heart disease. In our series, no patient underwent chemoembolisation.

IV.7.3.2. Radio frequency :

It is generally indicated for hepatic metastases up to 3 cm in size. It can be combined with surgical treatment, especially for metastases larger than 3 cm in diameter. None of our patients has been treated with radiofrequency.

IV.7.4. External radiotherapy :

Digestive NETs have often been considered radio-resistant, but radiotherapy can be effective for analgesic purposes in bone metastases and can even reduce liver and brain metastases [92].

IV.7.5. Endoscopic treatment :

It is of interest in gastric (Type 1 and 2) and rectal NETs whose size does not exceed 2 cm. Polypectomy or mucosectomy may be proposed in these cases. Onozato Y et al evaluated the endoscopic treatment of 40 rectal NETs; complete resection of the NET by polypectomy was achieved in only 20% of cases, whereas submucosal dissection enabled removal of the tumour in 77.8% of cases and no local or distant recurrence was reported [93]. In our series, two NETs were treated endoscopically: a rectal NET with incomplete resection requiring surgery. The NET recurred at a distant site (liver) after a median follow-up of 48 months; and a gastric NET in atrophic gastritis.

IV.7.6. Surgical treatment of non-metastatic NETs :

Surgery is the preferred treatment whenever possible. The surgical procedure will depend on the location of the tumour and the local extension assessment.

IV .7.6.1 Pre-operative preparation :

When major surgery is planned in patients with carcinoid syndrome, prophylactic treatment with somatostatin analogues should be considered. The recommended dose of octreotide is 50 micrograms/hour intravenously, initiated 12 hours before surgery and continued until 24 to 48 hours after surgery [94, 95].

Any drug that stimulates histamine secretion should be avoided peri-operatively [96].

V   V.7.62. Gastric NETs :

The surgical approach depends on the type of tumour.

Type 1 and 2 NETs that are larger than 1 cm without invasion of the muscularis or lymph node metastasis are treated endoscopically by mucosectomy. In the event of invasion of the muscularis or lymph node metastasis, tumour resection surgery or antrectomy is indicated. In exceptional cases, a total gastrectomy may be performed. For sporadic NETs (type 3), adenocarcinoma-type carcinological surgery is recommended [97].

In our series, a gastric NET was surgically resected. It was a mixed adenoneuroendocrine carcinoma.

VI .7.6.3. Duodeno-pancreatic NETs :

They form a specific group of tumours whose management will depend on the location of the tumour and the patient's background, and above all on whether or not they have NME1 [98, 99].

- **In the absence of NME1 :**

Surgical treatment is indicated even if the tumour is locally advanced, unless there is a high risk of post-operative mortality.

Insulinomas can be treated by enucleation provided that pathological examination confirms complete exeresis of the lesion and its benignity [100].

Non-enucleable G1 tumours < 2 cm in size located in the head of the pancreas can be monitored using MRI or CT.

- **In the presence of NME1 :**

In this case, tumours larger than 2 cm and increasing in size should be operated on, in the presence of adenopathy, and functional tumours (insulinoma, glucagonoma, Vipoma) [101].

For undifferentiated pancreatic NETs, surgery is only indicated for curative purposes [102]. A retrospective series of 108 patients with pancreatic NET with NEM1 concluded that survival rates were comparable between surgically treated and untreated patients [103].

In our series, 8 patients (2 ampullary and 6 pancreatic NETs) underwent surgical treatment: 4 cases of CPP and 4 caudal pancreatectomies.

IV.7.6.4. Gallic NETs :

Surgical resection of these tumours is indicated especially in cases of retractile mesenteritis, which is common in this condition. Even if there are hepatic metastases, resection of the primary site is indicated, to avoid complications such as occlusion or haemorrhage [102]. The entire graft must be explored, as these tumours are multiple in 20-30% of cases.

In our series, the 7 cases of grafted NET were surgically resected, two of which had hepatic metastases.

IV.7.6.5. Appendicular NETs :

They are usually operated on as an emergency measure in the event of an appendicular syndrome.

For NETs < 1 cm in size, appendectomy is sufficient. In a study published in 2014, Sarra E Murray et al concluded that there was no regional or distant recurrence of appendiceal NET < 1 cm treated with simple appendectomy [104]. This is consistent with data from other studies [105, 106] and with our series where none of the 17 patients with < 1cm NET (73.9%) recurred after a mean follow-up of 52.5 months.

A right hemicolectomy is indicated if the size is greater than 2 cm or in cases of Goblet cell carcinoid [107-109].

If the tumour size is between 1 and 2 cm, right hemicolectomy is indicated in the presence of one of these factors [110, 111]:

-Location at the base of the appendix

-Invasion of the meso-appendix of more than 3 mm

-Cellular atypia

-Venous or lymphatic emboli

-Neuroendocrine carcinomas.

IV.7.6.6. Colonic NETs :

Adenocarcinoma-type colectomy with lymph node dissection is indicated.

Surgery is indicated even in cases of local invasion or metastases, given the risk of complications such as occlusion or haemorrhage [112]. In our series, the only colonic NET was treated by right hemicolectomy with a recurrence-free survival of 3 months.

IV.7.6.7. Rectal NETs :

Treatment is guided by tumour size, deep invasion assessed by endoscopic ultrasound, degree of differentiation and mitotic index.

G1 lesions up to 1 cm in diameter are treated by endoscopic or trans-anal resection if there is no vascular or muscular invasion.

For tumours larger than 2 cm, radical carcinological surgery (adenocarcinoma) is recommended.

For tumours between 1 and 2 cm in size, either trans-anal resection or radical surgery is recommended depending on lymph node extension, vascular invasion and tumour grade (G1 or G2). According to Park et al, the predictive size for the presence of metastasis was greater than 1.4 cm [113]. Moore et al evaluated the results of endoscopic and surgical treatment of rectal NET in a retrospective series of 37 patients. Of the 35 patients (94.5%) with tumours smaller than 1 cm treated endoscopically (polypectomy or mucosectomy), 2 recurred (5.7%) [114].

In our series, one case of a 12 mm polypoid NET was treated by polypectomy with incomplete exeresis requiring additional anterior resection, and a 2eme case of a midrectal NET was treated by anterior resection.

IV.7.7. Treatment of well-differentiated hepatic metastases :

IV.7.7.1. Résécables :

Surgical resection of metastases or tumour destruction associated with resection of the primary tumour should always be discussed [115]. Unfortunately, radical treatment is only possible in less than 10% of patients [116]. The 5-year survival rate after resection of the primary tumour and metastasis can be as high as 74%, with a post-operative mortality rate of 6% [117, 118]. Diagram 3 illustrates the different therapeutic approaches to resectable, well-differentiated hepatic metastases [70].

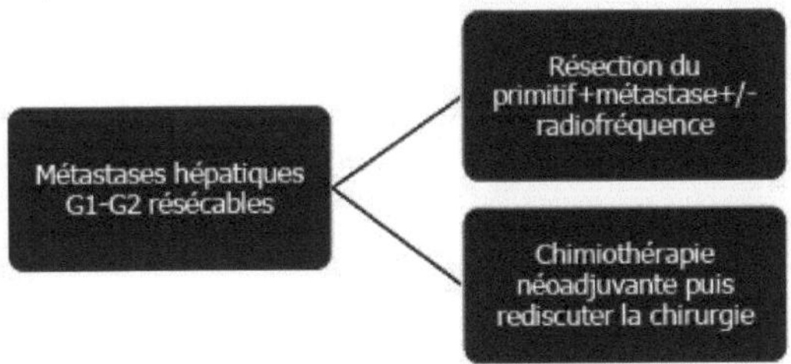

Diagram 3: Therapeutic options for resectable G1-G2 liver metastases

IV.7.7.2. Non-resectable :

Treatment depends on the location of the primary tumour and the histological characteristics of the tumour (Ki67, tumour size, etc.). Several therapeutic modalities can be proposed: somatostatin analogues, chemotherapy, targeted therapy, chemoembolisation or radiotherapy. Diagrams 4 and 5 show the different therapeutic options in the case of non-resectable hepatic metastases that are well differentiated from a duodeno-pancreatic or graft origin [70] :

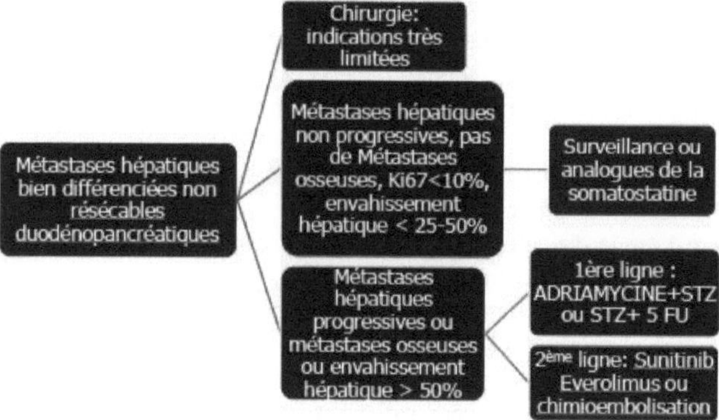

Diagram 4: Treatment of well-differentiated
non-resectable duodenopancreatic liver metastases
[70].

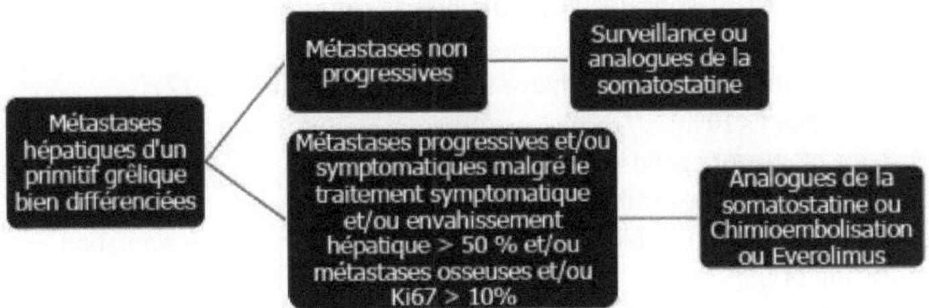

Diagram 5: Treatment of non-resectable liver metastases from a graft or other (non-pancreatic) primary site

In our series, hepatic metastases were not resectable in any case. Treatment with somatostatin analogues or chemotherapy was indicated.

Figure 6 illustrates the therapeutic algorithm for metastatic digestive NET, regardless of the site of the primary tumour [70].

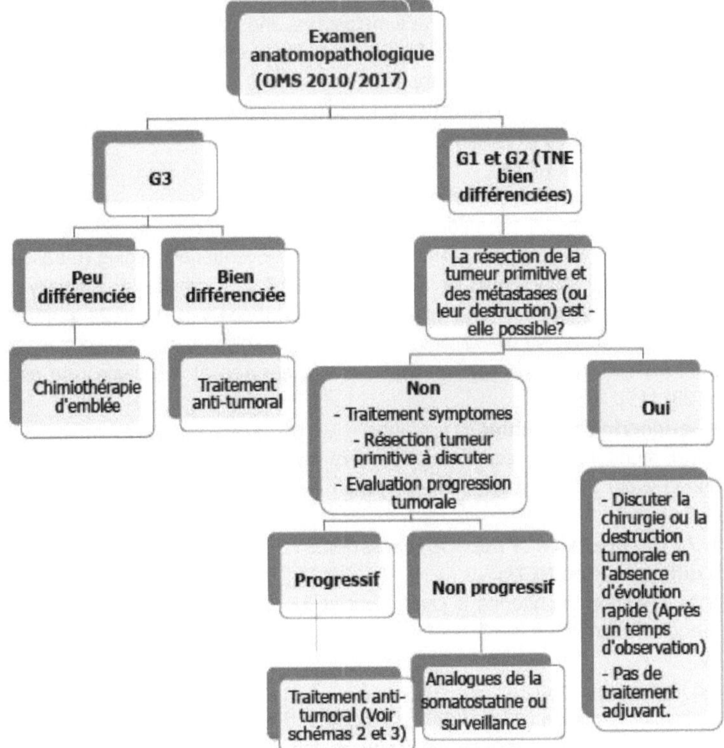

Schema 6: Management of metastatic digestive NET, regardless of the site of the primary tumour [70].

IV.7.7.3. Liver transplantation (TH) :

If all the above treatments fail, TH should be considered [119]. The 1-year recurrence-free survival after TH can be as high as 77% [120]. A multicentre French series of 85 patients who underwent TH for NET concluded that the 5-year recurrence-free survival rate was 20% [121].

A number of criteria must be met to achieve better results (ENETS 2012):

- A low Ki-67 index (<10%).
- The absence of extra-hepatic lesions.
- The primary tumour is resected or resectable.
- The patient must remain stable for at least 6 months prior to transplantation.
- Under the age of 55.
- Metastases occupy less than 50% of the liver.

None of our patients underwent TH for liver metastases.

IV.7.8. Post-therapeutic monitoring :

Surveillance of digestive NETs depends on three factors: the degree of differentiation, the distant extension of the tumour and the type of treatment initially instituted.

IV. 7.8.1. Situations requiring no monitoring :

Rectal NETs: well differentiated G1, less than 10 mm in size, no muscular involvement, no venous or lymphatic emboli, no lymph node metastases and completely resected.

Appendiceal NETs: well differentiated, G1, < 2 cm, base not affected by the tumour, no lymph node metastases in the meso-appendix, no venous or lymphatic emboli, no meso-invasion of more than 3 mm and non-adenocarcinoid in nature.

IV.7.8.2. In the absence of hepatic metastases :

- **Well differentiated NETs:**

Monitoring must be prolonged, for at least 10 years.

Surveillance intervals should be modulated according to prognostic factors (grade, stage, tumour volume, R0 or R1 resection). After R0 surgery, conventional imaging (ultrasound, CT or MRI) and an octreoscan should be repeated within 3 to 6 months if it initially showed lesions, then imaging every 6 to 12 months for 5 years, then every 12 to 24 months for 10 years, then every 5 years. No biological marker is valid for follow-up. It is recommended that chromogranin A and initially abnormal markers be measured at the same rate as clinical follow-up [25, 115].

- **Neuroendocrine carcinoma :**

Close clinical monitoring is recommended every two months. Imaging (CT or MRI) is recommended every 2 months for 6 months, then every 3 months for 1 year, then every 6 months.

IV.7.8.3. In the presence of hepatic metastases :

- **Well differentiated NETs:**

After hepatic resection: Monitoring is carried out at 3 months post-operatively with a CT or MRI scan and an octreoscan if initially positive, followed by a CT or MRI scan every 3 to 6 months.

Unresected liver metastases:

Monitoring involves imaging (CT or MRI) at 3 months, then every 3 to 6 months for 2 years, then every 6 to 12 months if the lesions remain stable. The value of regular octreoscans or PET scans, if initially positive, has not been proven, but is recommended by ENETS every 1 to 2 years. Cardiac ultrasound is recommended every 6 to 12 months to look for carcinoid cardiopathy in the event of carcinoid syndrome or elevation of urinary 5 HIAA.

Complications of treatment (chemotherapy, radiotherapy) should always be investigated [122].

- **Neuroendocrine carcinoma :**

A thoracic-abdominal-pelvic CT scan is recommended, initially every 2 months and then as the lesions progress [70].

IV.8. Prognosis :

The prognosis is variable and depends on several factors. The best 5-year survival rates reported by the SEER and NRC (table XIX) were noted in the rectal location (74 to 88%). Pancreatic NETs had a poorer prognosis, with a 5-year survival rate of 27-43% [5, 10]. A Tunisian study of 32 digestive NETs reported a 5-year survival of 62% [13].

Table XIX: 5-year survival of PNETs according to American and Norwegian registries

	SEER(USA)	NRC(Norway)	Our series
5-year survival (all sites)	64%	56%	**49%**

(SEER: Surveillance, Epidemiology and End Results; NRC: Norwegian Registry of Cancer)

The main prognostic factors are :

IV.8.1. Tumour size :

This is an important prognostic factor. A British retrospective series of 35 patients with gastrointestinal NETs concluded that there was a significant difference in the presence of lymph node and distant metastases between NETs < 1 cm and those > 1 cm [123]. Another study published in 2013 confirmed the significant increase in the risk of metastases for rectal NETs > 2 cm [124]. In our series, metastatic NETs had a mean size of 34 mm, and the rectal NET that recurred as hepatic metastasis had a size of 12 mm, which is consistent with the literature. Tumour size greater than 30 mm reduced survival in our patients, but the correlation was not significant (p=0.3).

IV.8.2. Histological grade :

Its prognostic value has been demonstrated by numerous studies [73, 125-127]. Jernman et al evaluated the prognostic contribution of tumour grade in rectal NETs and concluded that there was a significant difference in survival and presence of metastasis between G1 and G2 [71]. In our series, grades 2 or 3 had a poorer survival but no significant difference (p=0.1).

IV.8.3. Tumour differentiation :

Poorly differentiated tumours have a poor prognosis and are generally metastatic at diagnosis. Panzuto et al confirmed these results in a series of 185 patients with a GEP NET. The multivariate study isolated pancreatic location, distant metastases and low degree of differentiation as pejorative factors [11].

In our series, two tumours were poorly differentiated: one of graft origin with hepatic metastases, and the other 2eme was colonic with lymph node metastases. Our patients with a well-differentiated NET had significantly better survival (p<0.001).

IV.8.4. Tumour stage :

Tumour stage is a key prognostic factor. According to Pape UF et al, the 5-year survival for stages 1, 2 and 3 is 96%, 73% and 28% respectively [128]. Min Yang et al confirmed these results for pancreatic cancer, concluding that there was a significant difference in 5-year overall survival between the different stages [74]. In our series, there was no significant difference in survival between the different stages.

IV.8.5. Vascular invasion and metastatic character :

They worsen the prognosis; 90% of metastatic neuroendocrine tumours are accompanied by vascular emboli. Jernman et al concluded that mean survival was significantly reduced in the presence of vascular emboli in a retrospective series of 68 rectal NETs [71]. In our series, the presence of metastases significantly reduced the survival of our patients (p=0.07).

V CONCLUSIONS

56

Digestive neuroendocrine tumours are a rare group of tumours whose prevalence does not exceed 1 to 2% of all tumours. It is a heterogeneous group as the different clinical, morphological, therapeutic and especially prognostic aspects depend on multiple factors including site, grade and histological stage.

Their rarity and heterogeneity have made these tumours an interesting subject to study from an epidemiological and histological point of view, giving rise over the years to a multitude of classifications, most often incompletely validated, until the advent of the WHO 2010 classification, recently revised in 2017, which identifies 4 categories of NET based on histological and immunohistochemical criteria.

The complexity of these tumours has motivated our retrospective study, which consisted of evaluating their epidemiological, clinical, histological and therapeutic characteristics and highlighting the prognostic factors through the experience of a Tunisian gastroenterology and digestive surgery centre over a 12-year period from 2005 to 2016.

The mean age of our patients was 43.3 years, with a slight female predominance (sex ratio 0.85). Contrary to the literature, where graft location was found to be the most frequent, in our series, appendicular location was predominant in 41.8% of cases, followed by pancreatic location in 14.5% of cases, graft location in 12,7% of cases, one of which was associated with a mesenteric site, gastric in 6 cases (10.9%), duodenal in 3 cases (5.4%), primary mesenteric in 2 cases (3.6%), rectal in 2 cases (3.6%), colonic in 1 case, and hepatic metastases of an unknown primary in 3 cases. Primary mesenteric location is very rare, if not exceptional, as reported in case reports.

Clinical presentation, treatment modalities and course varied according to the site of the tumour.

For the stomach, abdominal pain was the most frequent diagnostic sign (100% of cases). EOGD is an essential examination in the diagnosis of gastric NETs; in our series, it was performed in all cases. Only one patient with mixed carcinoma had undergone surgical treatment in this location, consisting of subtotal gastrectomy. Mean survival in this location was 62 months.

Three cases of duodenal NET were reported in our series, two of which were ampullary. They were revealed by abdominal pain in all cases and vomiting in 2/3 of cases. Positive diagnosis was based on a combination of EOGD and abdominal CT. These two examinations enabled the diagnosis to be made in all 3 cases. Treatment consisted of a simple biopsy-exeresis for one bulbar millimetric NET and CPP for the two ampullary NETs. Mean survival was 19 months for this location. No tumour recurrence was noted.

Graft location accounted for 12.7% of all locations. The tumour was revealed by abdominal pain in 2/3 of cases and an occlusive syndrome in 1/3 of cases. Abdominal CT scans were used to make the diagnosis in 6 cases; they are the gold standard for this type of tumour and can even show atypical features that are highly suggestive of the diagnosis, such as fibrosis with retraction of the mesentery. The prognosis for grafted NETs is good, with the average survival of our patients being around 20 months.

NETs occupy 1[ere] place in terms of frequency for appendicular location; 42% of our patients had an appendicular tumour. The most frequent presentation was abdominal pain (100%). A carcinoid syndrome was observed in one patient. Most appendiceal NETs were discovered incidentally and were less than 1 cm in size. All our patients had undergone appendectomy and there was no recurrence in this location with a mean survival time of 50 months. No surveillance is required for appendiceal NETs measuring less than 10 mm, and their survival rate is similar to that of the general population.

The incidence of colorectal tumours was no more than 6%. The tumour was revealed by an occlusive syndrome in 1/3 of cases and rectal discharge in 1/3 of cases. Colonoscopy was the gold standard and led to a positive diagnosis in all cases. Mean survival for this location was 30 months. One patient operated for colonic NET died 3 months post-operatively. One patient operated for a rectal NET developed metachronous hepatic metastases after 48 months, which justifies regular and prolonged post-operative surveillance.

Eight cases of pancreatic NET were noted in our study. The most frequent presenting symptom was abdominal pain (100%) and AEG (75%). Abdominal CT is the gold standard for this location, and was diagnostic in all cases. Surgery is always indicated in the absence of NME 1 for non-metastatic NETs. In the case of hepatic metastases, treatment depends essentially on tumour grade, tumour volume and the presence or absence of extrahepatic sites. In our series, 6 patients underwent surgery: Q=four had undergone left pancreatectomy and two had undergone CPP. Mean survival was 11 months and

The course was marked by tumour progression on somatostatin analogues and subsequently on chemotherapy in one patient.

In 3 cases, no primary was found in patients with hepatic metastases. OCT scans were performed in all three patients.

Anatomopathologically, the diagnosis was made on biopsy in 15 cases (27.2%) and on operative specimen in 44 cases (80%). The mean size of the tumours was 19.65 mm. The majority of these tumours were well differentiated (92.7%), which is consistent with the literature. Microscopic examination was used to classify the tumours according to WHO 2010 recommendations, specifying the mitotic index and proliferation index, to specify the TNM stage according to UICC/AJCC 2009 (7eme edition), and to assess histological and prognostic factors.

The mean mitotic index was 3 mitoses/10 CFG. Immunohistochemistry is a cornerstone in the positive diagnosis and prognostic evaluation of these tumours. The most commonly used differentiation markers were chromogranin A, which was positive in 80% of cases, and synaptophysin, which was positive in 72.7% of cases. Ki67, a major prognostic factor, varied from 0 to 40% with an average of 5%. A correlation study between the proliferation index and tumour size showed a positive correlation (p=0.06). Thirty patients (54.5%) had grade 1 NET (G1), 21 (38.1%) had grade 2 NET (G2) and 2 patients had neuroendocrine carcinoma. Two patients in our series had mixed adeno-neuroendocrine carcinoma. The cases in our series were classified according to the UICC/AJCC 7 TNM stages^{eme} edition as follows: Stage 0: 1 case (1.8%), Stage I: 31 cases (56.3%), Stage IIA: 9 cases (16.3%), Stage IIB: 2 cases (3.6%), Stage IIIA: 1 case (1.8%), Stage IIIB: 2 cases (3.6%), Stage IV: 4 cases (7.2%), and unclassifiable tumour: 5 cases (9%).

Only one patient, operated for colonic NET, died after 3 months' follow-up. Eighteen patients were lost to follow-up after a mean of 28.2 months. The outcome was favourable in 32 cases (62%): 4 cases of gastric NET, 1 case of duodenal NET (ampullary), 5 cases of NET of the graft, 1 case of NET with dual graft and mesenteric localisation, 17 cases of appendicular NET, 3 cases of pancreatic NET and one case of primary mesenteric NET. Tumour progression was observed in 3 cases: a pancreatic NET with hepatic metastases that progressed under somatostatin analogues, an operated rectal NET that recurred as hepatic metastases and a mixed adenoneuroendocrine gastric carcinoma that progressed under post-operative chemotherapy.

Overall survival at 5 years in our patients was 49%. It was significantly better for appendicular, gall bladder and mesenteric sites than for colorectal and pancreatic sites (p=0.007). Two other parameters were associated with better survival in our patients: tumour differentiation and tumour size. Ki67, which is inversely correlated with survival in some studies, was not significantly correlated with survival in our series.

Tumour grade is a major prognostic factor, as demonstrated in a number of Italian and German studies. In our work, we found no significant correlation between grade and tumour stage. However, tumour size was significantly associated with grade.

Tumour stage was significantly associated with three histopronostic parameters: size, presence of metastases and vascular emboli.

Our study thus confirms the epidemioclinical heterogeneity of these tumours and their histological complexity, necessitating the use of regularly revised classifications (WHO, UICC).

From an epidemiological and clinical point of view, we have found that appendicular location, contrary to the classic data, is not so rare, which motivates a meticulous examination of any appendectomy specimen in search of a carcinoid tumour that may go unnoticed.

In terms of prognosis, our results confirm the limitations of the 2010 WHO classification, which was not significantly associated with tumour stage, whereas tumour size was positively correlated with tumour grade and stage. Therefore, other parameters for assessing tumour aggressiveness and malignancy, such as tumour site and size, should be evaluated in the new 2017 WHO classification, which is certainly more efficient but also seems to omit these two important histopronostic parameters.

In terms of surveillance, we recommend adapting the frequency of surveillance to each tumour site, given that the location of the tumour significantly affected survival in our series, with a guarded prognosis for pancreatic and colorectal sites.

VI REFERENCES

1. De Mestier L, Deguelte-Lardiere S, Brixi H, Kianmanesh R, Cadiot G. Digestive neuroendocrine tumors. Rev Med Interne. 2016;37(8):551-60.

2. Leotlela PD, Jauch A, Holtgreve-Grez H, Thakker RV. Genetics of neuroendocrine and carcinoid tumours. Endocr Relat Cancer. 2003;10(4):437-50.

3. Aloui S. Evaluation of histopronostic factors in neuroendocrine tumors of the digestive tract: A propos de 36 cas [These]. Medecine: Tunis; 2016. 81p.

4. Niederle MB, Hackl M, Kaserer K, Niederle B. Gastroenteropancreatic neuroendocrine tumours: the current incidence and staging based on the WHO and European Neuroendocrine Tumour Society classification: an analysis based on prospectively collected parameters. Endocr Relat Cancer. 2010;17(4):909-18.

5. Modlin IM, Lye KD, Kidd M. A 5-decade analysis of 13,715 carcinoid tumors. Cancer. 2003;97(4):934-59.

6. Yao JC, Hassan M, Phan A, Dagohoy C, Leary C, Mares JE, et al. One hundred years after "carcinoid": epidemiology of and prognostic factors for neuroendocrine tumors in 35,825 cases in the United States. J Clin Oncol. 2008;26(18):3063-72.

7. Bilimoria KY, Bentrem DJ, Wayne JD, Ko CY, Bennett CL, Talamonti MS. Small bowel cancer in the United States: changes in epidemiology, treatment, and survival over the last 20 years. Ann Surg. 2009;249(1):63-71.

8. Walter T, Lepage C. Epidemiology of digestive neuroendocrine tumours: the situation in France. Hepato Gastro. 2013;20:160-6.

9. Modlin IM, Champaneria MC, Chan AK, Kidd M. A three-decade analysis of 3,911 small intestinal neuroendocrine tumors: the rapid pace of no progress. Am J Gastroenterol. 2007;102(7):1464-73.

10. Hauso O, Gustafsson BI, Kidd M, Waldum HL, Drozdov I, Chan AK, et al. Neuroendocrine tumor epidemiology: contrasting Norway and North America. Cancer. 2008;113(10):2655-64.

11. Panzuto F, Nasoni S, Falconi M, Corleto VD, Capurso G, Cassetta S, et al. Prognostic factors and survival in endocrine tumor patients: comparison between gastrointestinal and pancreatic localization. Endocr Relat Cancer. 2005;12(4):1083-92.

12. Niederle MB, Niederle B. Diagnosis and treatment of gastroenteropancreatic neuroendocrine tumors: current data on a prospectively collected, retrospectively analyzed clinical multicenter investigation. Oncologist. 2011;16(5):602-13.

13. Larguech M. Les tumeurs neuroendocrines digestives a propos d'une serie de 32 cas [These]. Anatomopathologie: Tunis; 2013. 128p.

14. Ramage JK, Ahmed A, Ardill J, Bax N, Breen DJ, Caplin ME, et al. Guidelines for the management of gastroenteropancreatic neuroendocrine (including carcinoid) tumours (NETs). Gut. 2012;61(1):6-32.

15. Vinik AI, Woltering EA, Warner RR, Caplin M, O'Dorisio TM, Wiseman GA, et al. NANETS consensus guidelines for the diagnosis of neuroendocrine tumor. Pancreas. 2010;39(6):713-34.

16. Caplin ME, Buscombe JR, Hilson AJ, Jones AL, Watkinson AF, Burroughs AK. Carcinoid tumour. The Lancet. 1998;352(9130):799-805.

17. Pellikka PA, Tajik AJ, Khandheria BK, Seward JB, Callahan JA, Pitot HC, et al. Carcinoid heart disease. Clinical and echocardiographic spectrum in 74 patients. Circulation. 1993;87(4):1188-96.

18. Maru DM, Khurana H, Rashid A, Correa AM, Anandasabapathy S, Krishnan S, et al. Retrospective study of clinicopathologic features and prognosis of high-grade neuroendocrine carcinoma of the esophagus. Am J Surg Pathol. 2008;32(9):1404-11.

19. Modlin IM, Lye KD, Kidd M. Carcinoid tumors of the stomach. Surg Oncol. 2003;12(2):153-72.

20. Eriksson B, Kloppel G, Krenning E, Ahlman H, Plockinger U, Wiedenmann B, et al. Consensus guidelines for the management of patients with digestive neuroendocrine tumors. Neuroendocrinology. 2008;87(1):8-19.

21. Scherubl H, Jensen RT, Cadiot G, Stolzel U, Kloppel G. Neuroendocrine tumors of the small bowels are on the rise: Early aspects and management. World J Gastrointest Endosc. 2010;2(10):325-34.

22. Jensen RT, Cadiot G, Brandi ML, de Herder WW, Kaltsas G, Komminoth P, et al. ENETS Consensus Guidelines for the management of patients with digestive neuroendocrine neoplasms: functional pancreatic endocrine tumor syndromes. Neuroendocrinology. 2012;95(2):98-119.

23. Metz DC, Jensen RT. Gastrointestinal neuroendocrine tumors: pancreatic endocrine tumors. Gastroenterology. 2008;135(5):1469-92.

24. Hirabayashi K, Zamboni G, Nishi T, Tanaka A, Kajiwara H, Nakamura N. Histopathology of gastrointestinal neuroendocrine neoplasms. Front Oncol. 2013;3:2.

25. Caplin M, Sundin A, Nillson O, Baum RP, Klose KJ, Kelestimur F, et al. ENETS Consensus Guidelines for the management of patients with digestive neuroendocrine neoplasms: colorectal neuroendocrine neoplasms. Neuroendocrinology. 2012;95(2):88-97.

26. Kwaan MR, Goldberg JE, Bleday R. Rectal carcinoid tumors: review of results after endoscopic and surgical therapy. Arch Surg. 2008;143(5):471-5.

27. Oberg K. Biochemical diagnosis of neuroendocrine GEP tumor. Yale J Biol Med. 1997;70(5-6):501-8.

28. Frilling A, Modlin IM, Kidd M, Russell C, Breitenstein S, Salem R, et al. Recommendations for management of patients with neuroendocrine liver metastases. Lancet Oncol. 2014;15(1):8-21.

29. Seng-Kee Chuah T-HH, Chung-Mou Kuo, King-Wah Chiu, Chung-Huang Kuo, Keng-Liang Wu, Yeh-Pin Chou S-NL, Shue-Shian Chiou, Chi-Sin Changchien, Hock-Liew Eng. Upper gastrointestinal carcinoid tumors incidentally found by endoscopic examinations. World J Gastroenterol. 2005;11(44):7028-32.

30. Shim KN, Yang SK, Myung SJ, Chang HS, Jung SA, Choe JW, et al. Atypical endoscopic features of rectal carcinoids. Endoscopy. 2004;36(4):313-6.

31. Rondonotti E, Pennazio M, Toth E, Menchen P, Riccioni ME, De Palma GD, et al. Small-bowel neoplasms in patients undergoing video capsule endoscopy: a multicenter European study. Endoscopy. 2008;40(6):488-95.

32. Hara AK, Leighton JA, Sharma VK, Heigh RI, Fleischer DE. Imaging of small bowel disease: comparison of capsule endoscopy, standard endoscopy, barium examination, and CT. Radiographics. 2005;25(3):697-711.

33. Ganeshan D, Bhosale P, Yang T, Kundra V. Imaging features of carcinoid tumors of the gastrointestinal tract. Am J Roentgenol. 2013;201(4):773-86.

34. Pilleul F, Penigaud M, Milot L, Saurin JC, Chayvialle JA, Valette PJ. Possible smallbowel neoplasms: contrast-enhanced and water-enhanced multidetector CT enteroclysis. Radiology. 2006;241(3):796-801.

35. Massironi S, Conte D, Sciola V, Pirola L, Paggi S, Fraquelli M, et al. Contrast-enhanced ultrasonography in evaluating hepatic metastases from neuroendocrine tumours. Dig Liver Dis. 2010;42(9):635-41.

36. Bushnell DL, Baum RP. Standard imaging techniques for neuroendocrine tumors.

Endocrinol Metab Clin North Am. 2011;40(1):153-62.

37. Ichikawa T, Peterson MS, Federle MP, Baron RL, Haradome H, Kawamori Y, et al. Islet cell tumor of the pancreas: biphasic CT versus MR imaging in tumor detection. Radiology. 2000;216(1):163-71.

38. Owen NJ, Sohaib SA, Peppercorn PD, Monson JP, Grossman AB, Besser GM, et al. MRI of pancreatic neuroendocrine tumours. Br J Radiol. 2001;74(886):968-73.

39. Semelka RC, Custodio CM, Cem Balci N, Woosley JT. Neuroendocrine tumors of the pancreas: spectrum of appearances on MRI. J Magn Reson Imaging. 2000;11(2):141-8.

40. Thoeni RF, Mueller-Lisse UG, Chan R, Do NK, Shyn PB. Detection of small, functional islet cell tumors in the pancreas: selection of MR imaging sequences for optimal sensitivity. Radiology. 2000;214(2):483-90.

41. Reznek RH. CT/MRI of neuroendocrine tumours. Cancer Imaging. 2006;6:S163-77.

42. Sotoudehmanesh R, Hedayat A, Shirazian N, Shahraeeni S, Ainechi S, Zeinali F, et al. Endoscopic ultrasonography (EUS) in the localization of insulinoma. Endocrine. 2007;31(3):238-41.

43. Sundin A. Radiological and nuclear medicine imaging of gastroenteropancreatic neuroendocrine tumours. Best Pract Res Clin Gastroenterol. 2012;26(6):803-18.

44. Kwekkeboom DJ, Krenning EP, Scheidhauer K, Lewington V, Lebtahi R, Grossman A, et al. ENETS Consensus Guidelines for the Standards of Care in Neuroendocrine Tumors: somatostatin receptor imaging with (111)In-pentetreotide. Neuroendocrinology. 2009;90(2):184-9.

45. Reubi JC, Kvols LK, Waser B, Nagorney DM, Heitz PU, Charboneau JW, et al. Detection of somatostatin receptors in surgical and percutaneous needle biopsy samples of carcinoids and islet cell carcinomas. Cancer Res. 1990;50(18):5969-77.

46. De Herder WW, Hofland LJ, van der Lely AJ, Lamberts SW. Somatostatin receptors in gastroentero-pancreatic neuroendocrine tumours. Endocr Relat Cancer. 2003;10(4):451-8.

47. Squires MH, 3rd, Volkan Adsay N, Schuster DM, Russell MC, Cardona K, Delman KA, et al. Octreoscan Versus FDG-PET for Neuroendocrine Tumor Staging: A Biological Approach. Ann Surg Oncol. 2015;22(7):2295-301.

48. Binderup T, Knigge U, Loft A, Mortensen J, Pfeifer A, Federspiel B, et al. Functional imaging of neuroendocrine tumors: a head-to-head comparison of somatostatin receptor scintigraphy, 123I-MIBG scintigraphy, and 18F-FDG PET. J Nucl Med. 2010;51(5):704-12.

49. Illouz F, Sadoul JL, Rohmer V. Somatostatin receptor-based imaging and therapy of digestive endocrine tumors. Ann Endocrinol. 2010;71 Suppl 1:S3-S12.

50. Ait Lhachmi N. Digestive neuroendocrine tumours [These]. Medecine: Marrakesh; 2011. 212p.

51. Kloppel G. Classification and pathology of gastroenteropancreatic neuroendocrine neoplasms. Endocr Relat Cancer. 2011;18 Suppl 1:S1-S16.

52. Makhlouf HR, Burke AP, Sobin LH. Carcinoid tumors of the ampulla of Vater: a comparison with duodenal carcinoid tumors. Cancer. 1999;85(6):1241-9.

53. Cohen C, Heymann MF, Michenet P, Memeteau F, Saint-Marc O, Emy P, et al. Duodenal somatostatinomas associated with von Recklinghausen's neurofibromatosis. A propos of 2 cases. Ann Pathol. 2000;20(6):609-11.

54. Bornstein-Quevedo L, Gamboa-Dominguez A. Carcinoid tumors of the duodenum and ampulla of Vater: a clinicomorphologic, immunohistochemical, and cell kinetic comparison. Hum Pathol. 2001;32(11):1252-6.

55. Maggard MA, O'Connell JB, Ko CY. Updated population-based review of carcinoid

tumors. Ann Surg. 2004;240(1):117-22.

56. Stinner B, Rothmund M. Neuroendocrine tumours (carcinoids) of the appendix. Best Pract Res Clin Gastroenterol. 2005;19(5):729-38.

57. Jetmore AB, Ray JE, Gathright JB, McMullen KM, Hicks TC, Timmcke AE. Rectal carcinoids: the most frequent carcinoid tumor. Dis Colon Rectum. 1992;35(8):717-25.

58. Pinchot SN, Holen K, Sippel RS, Chen H. Carcinoid tumors. Oncologist. 2008;13(12):1255-69.

59. Klimstra DS. Pathology reporting of neuroendocrine tumors: essential elements for accurate diagnosis, classification, and staging. Semin Oncol. 2013;40(1):23-36.

60. Hijioka M, Ito T, Igarashi H, Fujimori N, Lee L, Nakamura T, et al. Serum chromogranin A is a useful marker for Japanese patients with pancreatic neuroendocrine tumors. Cancer Sci. 2014;105(11):1464-71.

61. Al-Khafaji B, Noffsinger AE, Miller MA, DeVoe G, Stemmermann GN, Fenoglio-Preiser C. Immunohistologic analysis of gastrointestinal and pulmonary carcinoid tumors. Hum Pathol. 1998;29(9):992-9.

62. Rindi G, Kloppel G, Alhman H, Caplin M, Couvelard A, de Herder WW, et al. TNM staging of foregut (neuro)endocrine tumors: a consensus proposal including a grading system. Virchows Arch. 2006;449(4):395-401.

63. Capelli P, Fassan M, Scarpa A. Pathology grading and staging of GEP-NETs. Best Pract Res Clin Gastroenterol. 2012;26(6):705-17.

64. Couvelard A. Ki67 and neuroendocrine tumors. Ann Pathol. 2011;31 Suppl 5:S55-S6.

65. Strosberg J, Nasir A, Coppola D, Wick M, Kvols L. Correlation between grade and prognosis in metastatic gastroenteropancreatic neuroendocrine tumors. Hum Pathol. 2009;40(9):1262-8.

66. Khan MS, Luong TV, Watkins J, Toumpanakis C, Caplin ME, Meyer T. A comparison of Ki-67 and mitotic count as prognostic markers for metastatic pancreatic and midgut neuroendocrine neoplasms. Br J Cancer. 2013;108(9):1838-45.

67. Flejou JF. WHO Classification of digestive tumors: the fourth edition. Ann Pathol. 2011;31 Suppl 5:S27-31.

68. Strosberg JR, Cheema A, Weber J, Han G, Coppola D, Kvols LK. Prognostic validity of a novel American Joint Committee on Cancer Staging Classification for pancreatic neuroendocrine tumors. J Clin Oncol. 2011;29(22):3044-9.

69. Scoazec JY, Couvelard A, pour le reseau T. The new WHO classification of digestive neuroendocrine tumors. Ann Pathol. 2011;31(2):88-92.

70. Cadiot G, Baudin E, Coriat R, Couvelard A, de Mestier L, Dromain C, et al. "Neuroendocrine tumours". Thesaurus National de Cancerologie Digestive, 12-10-2017, [Online] http://www.tncd.org.

71. Jernman J, Valimaki MJ, Louhimo J, Haglund C, Arola J. The novel WHO 2010 classification for gastrointestinal neuroendocrine tumours correlates well with the metastatic potential of rectal neuroendocrine tumours. Neuroendocrinology. 2012;95(4):317-24.

72. Edge SB, Compton CC. The American Joint Committee on Cancer: the 7th edition of the AJCC cancer staging manual and the future of TNM. Ann Surg Oncol. 2010;17(6):1471-4.

73. Scarpa A, Mantovani W, Capelli P, Beghelli S, Boninsegna L, Bettini R, et al. Pancreatic endocrine tumors: improved TNM staging and histopathological grading permit a clinically efficient prognostic stratification of patients. Mod Pathol. 2010;23(6):824-33.

74. Yang M, Zeng L, Zhang Y, Wang WG, Wang L, Ke NW, et al. TNM staging of pancreatic neuroendocrine tumors: an observational analysis and comparison by both AJCC and ENETS

systems from 1 single institution. Medicine. 2015;94(12):660.

75. Araujo PB, Cheng S, Mete O, Serra S, Morin E, Asa SL, et al. Evaluation of the WHO 2010 grading and AJCC/UICC staging systems in prognostic behavior of intestinal neuroendocrine tumors. PLoS One. 2013;8(4):61538.

76. Colonoscopy Study Group of Korean Society of C. Clinical characteristics of colorectal carcinoid tumors. J Korean Soc Coloproctol. 2011;27(1):17-20.

77. Baudin E, Caron P, Lombard-Bohas C, Tabarin A, Mitry E, Reznick Y, et al. Malignant insulinoma: recommendations for workup and treatment. Presse Med. 2014;6 Suppl 1:S645-S59.

78. Rinke A, Muller HH, Schade-Brittinger C, Klose KJ, Barth P, Wied M, et al. Placebo-controlled, double-blind, prospective, randomized study on the effect of octreotide LAR in the control of tumor growth in patients with metastatic neuroendocrine midgut tumors: a report from the PROMID Study Group. J Clin Oncol. 2009;27(28):4656-63.

79. Tiensuu Janson EM, Ahlstrom H, Andersson T, Oberg KE. Octreotide and interferon alfa: a new combination for the treatment of malignant carcinoid tumours. Eur J Cancer. 1992;28A(10):1647-50.

80. Kolby L, Persson G, Franzen S, Ahren B. Randomized clinical trial of the effect of interferon alpha on survival in patients with disseminated midgut carcinoid tumours. Br J Surg. 2003;90(6):687-93.

81. Plockinger U, Wiedenmann B. Neuroendocrine tumors. Biotherapy. Best Pract Res Clin Endocrinol Metab. 2007;21(1):145-62.

82. Raymond E, Dahan L, Raoul JL, Bang YJ, Borbath I, Lombard-Bohas C, et al. Sunitinib malate for the treatment of pancreatic neuroendocrine tumors. N Engl J Med. 2011;364(6):501-13.

83. Pavel ME, Hainsworth JD, Baudin E, Peeters M, Horsch D, Winkler RE, et al. Everolimus plus octreotide long-acting repeatable for the treatment of advanced neuroendocrine tumours associated with carcinoid syndrome (RADIANT-2): a randomised, placebo-controlled, phase 3 study. Lancet. 2011;378(9808):2005-12.

84. Boussaha T, Rougier P, Taieb J, Lepere C. Digestive neuroendocrine tumors (DNET): the era of targeted therapies. Clin Res Hepatol Gastroenterol. 2013;37(2):134-41.

85. Walter T, Brixi-Benmansour H, Lombard-Bohas C, Cadiot G. New treatment strategies in advanced neuroendocrine tumours. Dig Liver Dis. 2012;44(2):95-105.

86. Dahan L, Bonnetain F, Rougier P, Raoul JL, Gamelin E, Etienne PL, et al. Phase III trial of chemotherapy using 5-fluorouracil and streptozotocin compared with interferon alpha for advanced carcinoid tumors: FNCLCC-FFCD 9710. Endocr Relat Cancer. 2009;16(4):1351- 61.

87. Pavel M, O'Toole D, Costa F, Capdevila J, Gross D, Kianmanesh R, et al. ENETS Consensus Guidelines Update for the Management of Distant Metastatic Disease of Intestinal, Pancreatic, Bronchial Neuroendocrine Neoplasms (NEN) and NEN of Unknown Primary Site. Neuroendocrinology. 2016;103(2):172-85.

88. Carrasco CH, Chuang VP, Wallace S. Apudomas metastatic to the liver: treatment by hepatic artery embolization. Radiology. 1983;149(1):79-83.

89. Ajani JA, Carrasco CH, Charnsangavej C, Samaan NA, Levin B, Wallace S. Islet cell tumors metastatic to the liver: effective palliation by sequential hepatic artery embolization. Ann Intern Med. 1988;108(3):340-4.

90. Kim YH, Ajani JA, Carrasco CH, Dumas P, Richli W, Lawrence D, et al. Selective hepatic arterial chemoembolization for liver metastases in patients with carcinoid tumor or islet cell carcinoma. Cancer Invest. 1999;17(7):474-8.

91. Hajarizadeh H, Ivancev K, Mueller CR, Fletcher WS, Woltering EA. Effective palliative treatment of metastatic carcinoid tumors with intra-arterial chemotherapy/chemoembolization combined with octreotide acetate. Am J Surg. 1992;163(5):479-83.

92. Chakravarthy A, Abrams RA. Radiation therapy in the management of patients with malignant carcinoid tumors. Cancer. 1995;75(6):1386-90.

93. Onozato Y, Kakizaki S, Iizuka H, Sohara N, Mori M, Itoh H. Endoscopic treatment of rectal carcinoid tumors. Dis Colon Rectum. 2010;53(2):169-76.

94. Roy RC, Carter RF, Wright PD. Somatostatin, anaesthesia, and the carcinoid syndrome. Peri-operative administration of a somatostatin analogue to suppress carcinoid tumour activity. Anaesthesia. 1987;42(6):627-32.

95. Pederzoli P, Falconi M, Bonora A, Salvia R, Sartori N, Contro C, et al. Cytoreductive surgery in advanced endocrine tumours of the pancreas. Ital J Gastroenterol Hepatol. 1999;31 Suppl 2:S207-12.

96. Dougherty TB, Cronau LH, Jr. Anesthetic implications for surgical patients with endocrine tumors. Int Anesthesiol Clin. 1998;36(3):31-44.

97. Delle Fave G, Kwekkeboom DJ, Van Cutsem E, Rindi G, Kos-Kudla B, Knigge U, et al. ENETS Consensus Guidelines for the management of patients with gastroduodenal neoplasms. Neuroendocrinology. 2012;95(2):74-87.

98. Bloomston M, Muscarella P, Shah MH, Frankel WL, Al-Saif O, Martin EW, et al. Cytoreduction results in high perioperative mortality and decreased survival in patients undergoing pancreatectomy for neuroendocrine tumors of the pancreas. J Gastrointest Surg. 2006;10(10):1361-70.

99. Teh SH, Deveney C, Sheppard BC. Aggressive pancreatic resection for primary pancreatic neuroendocrine tumor: is it justifiable? Am J Surg. 2007;193(5):610-3.

100. Kaczirek K, Ba-Ssalamah A, Schima W, Niederle B. The importance of preoperative localisation procedures in organic hyperinsulinism-experience in 67 patients. Wien Klin Wochenschr. 2004;116(11-12):373-8.

101. Falconi M, Bartsch DK, Eriksson B, Kloppel G, Lopes JM, O'Connor JM, et al. ENETS Consensus Guidelines for the management of patients with digestive neuroendocrine neoplasms of the digestive system: well-differentiated pancreatic non-functioning tumors. Neuroendocrinology. 2012;95(2):120-34.

102. Boudreaux JP. Surgery for gastroenteropancreatic neuroendocrine tumors (GEPNETS). Endocrinol Metab Clin North Am. 2011;40(1):163-71.

103. Triponez F, Dosseh D, Goudet P, Cougard P, Bauters C, Murat A, et al. Epidemiology data on 108 MEN 1 patients from the GTE with isolated nonfunctioning tumors of the pancreas. Ann Surg. 2006;243(2):265-72.

104. Murray SE, Lloyd RV, Sippel RS, Chen H, Oltmann SC. Postoperative surveillance of small appendiceal carcinoid tumors. Am J Surg. 2014;207(3):342-5.

105. Mullen JT, Savarese DM. Carcinoid tumors of the appendix: a population-based study. J Surg Oncol. 2011;104(1):41-4.

106. Roggo A, Wood WC, Ottinger LW. Carcinoid tumors of the appendix. Ann Surg. 1993;217(4):385-90.

107. Toumpanakis C, Standish RA, Baishnab E, Winslet MC, Caplin ME. Goblet cell carcinoid tumors (adenocarcinoid) of the appendix. Dis Colon Rectum. 2007;50(3):315-22.

108. Safioleas MC, Moulakakis KG, Kontzoglou K, Stamoulis J, Nikou GC, Toubanakis C, et al. Carcinoid tumors of the appendix. Prognostic factors and evaluation of indications for

right hemicolectomy. Hepatogastroenterology. 2005;52(61):123-7.

109.	O'Donnell ME, Carson J, Garstin WI. Surgical treatment of malignant carcinoid tumours of the appendix. Int J Clin Pract. 2007;61(3):431-7.

110.	Varisco B, McAlvin B, Dias J, Franga D. Adenocarcinoid of the appendix: is right hemicolectomy necessary? A meta-analysis of retrospective chart reviews. Am Surg. 2004;70(7):593-9.

111.	Bucher P, Gervaz P, Ris F, Oulhaci W, Egger JF, Morel P. Surgical treatment of appendiceal adenocarcinoid (goblet cell carcinoid). World J Surg. 2005;29(11):1436-9.

112.	Bernick PE, Klimstra DS, Shia J, Minsky B, Saltz L, Shi W, et al. Neuroendocrine carcinomas of the colon and rectum. Dis Colon Rectum. 2004;47(2):163-9.

113.	Park CH, Cheon JH, Kim JO, Shin JE, Jang BI, Shin SJ, et al. Criteria for decision making after endoscopic resection of well-differentiated rectal carcinoids with regard to potential lymphatic spread. Endoscopy. 2011;43(9):790-5.

114.	Moore JR, Greenwell B, Nuckolls K, Schammel D, Schisler N, Schammel C, et al. Neuroendocrine tumors of the rectum: a 10-year review of management. Am Surg. 2011;77(2):198-200.

115.	Frilling A, Akerstrom G, Falconi M, Pavel M, Ramos J, Kidd M, et al. Neuroendocrine tumor disease: an evolving landscape. Endocr Relat Cancer. 2012;19(5):163-85.

116.	Mayo SC, de Jong MC, Pulitano C, Clary BM, Reddy SK, Gamblin TC, et al. Surgical management of hepatic neuroendocrine tumor metastasis: results from an international multi-institutional analysis. Ann Surg Oncol. 2010;17(12):3129-36.

117.	Chamberlain RS, Canes D, Brown KT, Saltz L, Jarnagin W, Fong Y, et al. Hepatic neuroendocrine metastases: does intervention alter outcomes? J Am Coll Surg. 2000;190(4):432-45.

118.	Eriksson J, Stalberg P, Nilsson A, Krause J, Lundberg C, Skogseid B, et al. Surgery and radiofrequency ablation for treatment of liver metastases from midgut and foregut carcinoids and endocrine pancreatic tumors. World J Surg. 2008;32(5):930-8.

119.	Schweizer RT, Alsina AE, Rosson R, Bartus SA. Liver transplantation for metastatic neuroendocrine tumors. Transplant Proc. 1993;25(2):1973.

120.	Van Vilsteren FG, Baskin-Bey ES, Nagorney DM, Sanderson SO, Kremers WK, Rosen CB, et al. Liver transplantation for gastroenteropancreatic neuroendocrine cancers: Defining selection criteria to improve survival. Liver Transpl. 2006;12(3):448-56.

121.	Le Treut YP, Gregoire E, Belghiti J, Boillot O, Soubrane O, Mantion G, et al. Predictors of long-term survival after liver transplantation for metastatic endocrine tumors: an 85-case French multicentric report. Am J Transplant. 2008;8(6):1205-13.

122.	Pavel M, Baudin E, Couvelard A, Krenning E, Oberg K, Steinmuller T, et al. ENETS Consensus Guidelines for the management of patients with liver and other distant metastases from neuroendocrine neoplasms of foregut, midgut, hindgut, and unknown primary. Neuroendocrinology. 2012;95(2):157-76.

123.	Dronamraju SS, Joypaul VB. Management of gastrointestinal carcinoid tumours - 10 years experience at a district general hospital. J Gastrointest Oncol. 2012;3(2):120-9.

124.	Weinstock B, Ward SC, Harpaz N, Warner RR, Itzkowitz S, Kim MK. Clinical and prognostic features of rectal neuroendocrine tumors. Neuroendocrinology. 2013;98(3):180-7.

125.	Dhall D, Mertens R, Bresee C, Parakh R, Wang HL, Li M, et al. Ki-67 proliferative index predicts progression-free survival of patients with well-differentiated ileal neuroendocrine tumors. Hum Pathol. 2012;43(4):489-95.

126.	Jann H, Roll S, Couvelard A, Hentic O, Pavel M, Muller-Nordhorn J, et al.

Neuroendocrine tumors of midgut and hindgut origin: tumor-node-metastasis classification determines clinical outcome. Cancer. 2011;117(15):3332-41.

127. Panzuto F, Boninsegna L, Fazio N, Campana D, Pia Brizzi M, Capurso G, et al. Metastatic and locally advanced pancreatic endocrine carcinomas: analysis of factors associated with disease progression. J Clin Oncol. 2011;29(17):2372-7.

128. Pape UF, Jann H, Muller-Nordhorn J, Bockelbrink A, Berndt U, Willich SN, et al. Prognostic relevance of a novel TNM classification system for upper gastroenteropancreatic neuroendocrine tumors. Cancer. 2008;113(2):256-65.

VII APPENDICES

Appendix 1: Patient information sheet

Patient information sheet

- Age and sex
- Personal medical, surgical and family history
- History of NME1
- Circumstances of discovery
- Tumour site
- Standard biological tests (blood glucose, haemoglobin, inflammatory syndrome) and specific tests (urinary chromogranin A and 5 HIAA)
- Radiological and endoscopic examinations
- Anatomopathological examination: mitotic index, Ki67, lymph node invasion, etc.
- Tumour grade
- Tumour stage according to UICC/AJCC 7ᵉᵐᵉ edition
- Presence of metastases
- Therapeutic management
- Evolution and survival in months

Appendix 2: The tumour grade proposed by ENETS

Grade	Mitotic index (/10 CFG)	Proliferation index (%)
G1	<2	≤2
G2	2-20	3-20
G3	>20	>20

Appendix 3: WHO classification 2010

G1 neuroendocrine tumour	• Well differentiated tumour • Mitotic index < 2 • Ki-67 < 2%
G2 neuroendocrine tumour	• Well differentiated tumour • Mitotic index: 2-20 • Ki-67: 3 - 20
	• Poorly differentiated carcinoma • Mitotic index > 20 • Ki-67 > 20%
Neuroendocrine carcinoma: small/large cells **Mixed adeno-neuroendocrine carcinoma (MANEC)**	

Appendix 4 (A, B, C): TNM classification of digestive NCTs according to UICC/AJCC 7®ᵐᵉ edition

(A)	Stomach	Large intestine	Pancreas	Appendix	Colon/rectum
Tx	Non-evaluable tumour				
T0	No identifiable tumour				
Tis	T<5mm	NA	Carcinoma in situ	NA	NA
T1	Tumour invades lamina propria or	T invades mucosa or submucosa and T<	T limited to the pancreas and T<	T < or =2cm (T1a: < or	T invades the mucosa or sub-mucosa (T1a <

	sub-mucosa and T< or = 1cm	or = 1 cm	or = 2cm	=2cm) 1 cm; T1b: > 1-2 cm)	1cm; T1b: 1-2 cm)
T2	T invades muscularis or subserosa or T> 1cm	T invades muscularis or T>1cm	T limited to the pancreas and T> 2cm	T invades the cecum or T > 2-4 cm	T invades the muscularis or T>2cm
T3	T invades sereuse	T invades pancreas or retro-peritoneum (duodenum, ampulla)/ T invades sub-serosa (ileon, jejunum)	T extends beyond the pancreas but does not invade the cffiliac axis or the superior mesenteric artery	T invades the ileum or T> 4 cm	T invades the subserosa or pericolic/rectal fat
T4	T invades adjacent organs	T invades peritoneum or adjacent organs	T invades the cffiliac axis or the superior mesenteric artery	T invades the peritoneum or adjacent organs	T invades the peritoneum or adjacent organs

NX: status not assessable
NO: absence of lymph node metastasis
N1: presence of lymph node metastases

Ea^a§tastasesiai^

MX: status not assessable
MO: absence of distant metastasis
MI: presence of distant metastases

Appendix 5: UICC TNM classification 8eme edition

	Stomach	Vater/Duodenum ampoule	Grele intestine	Pancreas	Appendix	Colon/Rectum
Tx	Non-evaluable tumour					
T0	No identifiable tumour					
T1	T Involves lamina propria or submucosa and T < or = 1 cm	T invades the mucosa or submucosa and T<1cm (duodenal T) T<1cm and confined to the sphincter of Oddi (ampullary T)	T invades lamina propria or sub-mucosa and T < or = 1 cm	T limited to pancreas < 2 cm	T<2 cm	T invades mucosa or submucosa (T1a: <1 cm, T1b: 1-2 cm)
T2	T invades muscularis or T >1 cm	T invades muscularis or T>1 cm (duodenal T) /T infiltrates submucosa or duodenal muscularis	T invades muscularis or T>1 cm	T limited to pancreas, 24 cm	T >2-4 cm	T invades muscularis or T>2 cm with invasion of the mucosa or submucosa
T3	T invades sub serous	T invades pancreas or peripancreatic adipose tissue	T invades the sub-serosa (respects the serosa)	T limited to pancreas, >4 cm; or invades duodenum or choledochus	T >4 cm or T infiltrates subserosa or mesoappendix	T invades sub serous
T4	T invades the peritoneum or adjacent organs/structures	T invades peritoneum or other organs	T invades the serosa or other adjacent organs/structures	T invades adjacent organs (stomach, spleen, colon, suprarenal) or large vessels (cffiliac axis or superior mesenteric artery)	T perforates the peritoneum or infiltrates adjacent organs (except adjacent tube)	T invades peritoneum or adjacent organs/structures

Appendix 6: Clinical stages (All tumours except appendix and pancreas)

Stade	T	N M
0	Tis	N0M0
I	T1	N0M0
II a	T2	N0M0
II b	T3	N0M0
III a	T4	N0M0
III b	Tout T	N1M0
IV	Tout T	Tout N M1

Annex 7: Clinical stages (Appendix)

Stade	T	N M
I	T1	N0M0
II	T2, T3	N0M0
III	T4	N0M0
	Tout T	N1M0
IV	Tout T	Tout N M1

Appendix 8: Clinical stages (Pancreas)

Stadium	T	N M
0	Tis	N0M0
I	T1	N0M0
II a	T2	N0M0
II b	T3	N0M0
III a	Tl, T2, T3	N1M0
III b	T4	All N M0
IV	All T	All N M1

More
Books!

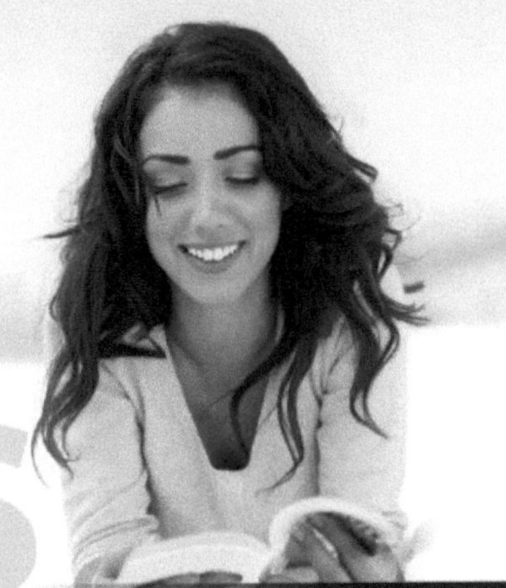

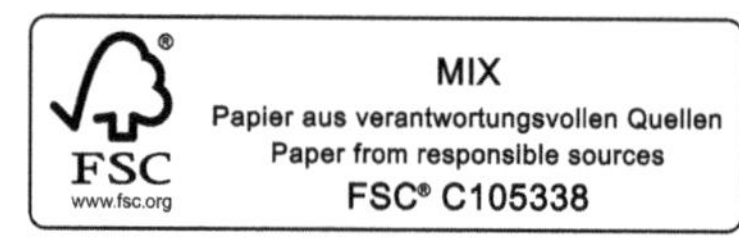

Printed by Books on Demand GmbH, Norderstedt / Germany